# Breast Cytopathology

# Syed Z. Ali, MD

Department of Pathology, The Johns Hopkins Hospital,
Baltimore, Maryland

# Anil V. Parwani, MD, PhD

Department of Pathology, UPMC Shadyside Hospital,
Pittsburgh, Pennsylvania

# Breast Cytopathology

With Contributions by
Maureen F. Zakowski, MD
and Edi Brogi, MD, PhD

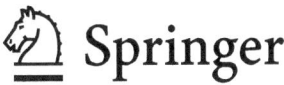 Springer

Syed Z. Ali, MD
Associate Professor of Pathology
  and Radiology
Associate Director, Cytopathology
  Fellowship Program
Department of Pathology
The Johns Hopkins Hospital
Baltimore, MD 21287
USA

Anil V. Parwani, MD, PhD
Assistant Professor of Pathology
Department of Pathology
UPMC Shadyside Hospital
Pittsburgh, PA 15232
USA

Series Editor
Dorothy L. Rosenthal, MD, FIAC
Professor of Pathology, Oncology, and Gynecology and Obstetrics
The Johns Hopkins Medical Institutions
Baltimore, MD 21287
USA

Library of Congress Control Number: 2007923714

ISBN: 978-0-387-71594-0          e-ISBN: 978-0-387-71595-7

Printed on acid-free paper.

9 8 7 6 5 4 3 2 1

springer.com

To my parents
Gul Bano (late) and Mazhar Ali
*Syed Z. Ali*


To my family
Namrata, Simran, Varun, and Sanam
*Anil V. Parwani*

# Foreword

This fourth volume in the series *Essentials in Cytopathology* revitalizes a topic that was considered headed for obsolescence a few years ago. Breast aspiration cytopathology was quickly being replaced by radiographically directed core biopsies. A major reason for this paradigm shift was the inability of breast fine-needle aspirates to predict the presence or absence of invasion in nonpalpable lesions.

However, as discussed in the following pages, there are multiple functions of a fine-needle aspirate beyond defining and staging a patient's primary lesion. Determining definite presence of metastases and recurrences is far more reliable by fine-needle aspiration than by imaging techniques, although the paired capabilities of imaging and aspiration can more accurately sample suspicious lesions than either technique alone.

On the horizon are molecular and genetic tests that will be based on samples obtained by fine-needle aspiration. Establishment of risk and tailored therapies will evolve from these descriptors of the natural history of a neoplastic process. After a half century of flat line progress against breast cancer, fine-needle aspiration will predictably play a major role in identifying personal risk factors and thereby controlling this lethal disease.

The authors bring combined expertise from major cancer centers where breast fine-needle aspiration is still utilized for patient management. Their experiences are now available in this volume to rejuvenate the skills of cytopathologists and raise their awareness of the true potential of breast fine-needle aspiration. I hope you appreciate their efforts and spread the word to your colleagues.

*Dorothy L. Rosenthal, MD, FIAC*
Baltimore, MD

# Series Preface

The subspecialty of cytopathology is 60 years old and has become established as a solid and reliable discipline in medicine. As expected, cytopathology literature has expanded in a remarkably short period of time, from a few textbooks prior to the 1980s to a current library of texts and journals devoted exclusively to cytomorphology that is substantial. *Essentials in Cytopathology* does not presume to replace any of the distinguished textbooks in cytopathology. Instead, the series will publish generously illustrated and user-friendly guides for both pathologists and clinicians.

Building on the amazing success of *The Bethesda System for Reporting Cervical Cytology*, now in its second edition, the series will utilize a similar format, including minimal text, tabular criteria, and superb illustrations based on real-life specimens. *Essentials in Cytopathology* will, at times, deviate from the classic organization of pathology texts. The logic of decision trees, elimination of unlikely choices, and narrowing of differential diagnosis via a pragmatic approach based on morphologic criteria are some of the strategies used to illustrate principles and practice in cytopathology.

Most of the authors for *Essentials in Cytopathology* are faculty members in The Johns Hopkins University School of Medicine, Department of Pathology, Division of Cytopathology. They bring to each volume the legacy of John K. Frost and the collective experience of a preeminent cytopathology service. The archives at Hopkins are meticulously catalogued and form the framework for text and illustrations. Authors from other institutions have been selected on the basis of their national reputations, experience, and enthusiasm for cytopathology. They bring to the series complimentary viewpoints and enlarge the scope of materials contained in the photographs.

The editor and authors are indebted to our students, past and future, who challenge and motivate us to become the best that we possibly can be. We share that experience with you through these pages and hope that you will learn from them as we have from those who have come before us. We would be remiss if we did not pay tribute to our professional colleagues, the cytotechnologists and preparatory technicians who lovingly care for the specimens that our clinical colleagues send to us.

Finally, we cannot emphasize enough throughout these volumes the importance of collaboration with the patient care team. Every specimen comes to us as a question begging an answer. Without input from the clinicians, complete patient history, results of imaging studies and other ancillary tests, we cannot perform optimally. It is our responsibility to educate our clinicians about their role in our interpretation and to integrate as much information as we can gather into our final diagnosis, even if the answer at first seems obvious.

We hope you will find this series useful and welcome your feedback as you place these handbooks by your microscopes and into your bookbags.

*Dorothy L. Rosenthal, MD, FIAC*
Baltimore, MD
July 15, 2004

# Preface

The study of breast disease by fine-needle aspiration, although diagnostically challenging, is a satisfying experience when accomplished properly, accurately, and as part of a team effort along with the radiologists and surgeons. Despite the upheavals that breast cytopathology has seen over the past decade with the advent of automated tissue biopsy devices, the procedure still plays an important role in most aspiration cytology laboratories, not only in major academic centers but also in many community-based practices. The spectrum of breast disease from nonneoplastic entities and pseudotumors to benign and malignant neoplasms is fascinating. Accurate interpretation requires careful evaluation of the often subtle cytologic characteristics but more likely hinges on a solid appreciation of the architectural appearance of the tissue fragments. Therefore, it goes without saying that for breast cytopathology, the interpreter requires knowledge and experience in the histopathology of breast disease.

Currently, there are a number of good texts available on cytopathology of the breast. However, in this book, the authors present their combined experience from three major U.S. teaching institutions (Johns Hopkins, University of Pittsburgh, and Memorial Sloan-Kettering Cancer Center) in a novel fashion: concise, methodical, and practical. The text has been kept to a minimum with only practical points of diagnostic importance. Differential diagnoses and pitfalls are included in an easy to read format. A generous number of carefully selected high-resolution images reinforce the key morphologic characteristics of the lesions discussed, enriching the reader's concepts. This book is morphology based and is intended for anyone who interprets breast cytopathology, from trainees in pathology to cytotechnologists to more experienced cytopathologists. Similar to the other books in the series, the basic approach is to use this as a "handbook," a readily available and user-friendly reference for quick consultations available by the side of the microscope in daily diagnostic work.

Finally, the authors would like to acknowledge the tremendous help and assistance provided to us by Mrs. Frances Burroughs, education coordinator and director of the school of cytotechnology at Hopkins. Fran was instrumental in selecting just the right glass slide cases for us to digitize from an enormous collection of study sets at Hopkins. We are also indebted to Dr. Dorothy Rosenthal for her invaluable feedback and suggestions to further enhance the usefulness of this book. Last but not least, our appreciation and thanks to the residents and fellows, who were the major motivation and impetus for writing this book.

*Syed Z. Ali, MD*
*Anil V. Parwani, MD, PhD*
Baltimore, MD

# Special Acknowledgment

The authors wish to express their gratitude to the following for their valuable contribution to the book:

*Maureen F. Zakowski, MD*
Attending Pathologist
Department of Pathology
Memorial Sloan-Kettering Cancer Center
New York, NY 10021
USA

*Edi Brogi, MD, PhD*
Assistant Attending Pathologist
Department of Pathology
Memorial Sloan-Kettering Cancer Center
New York, NY 10021
USA

# Contents

# 1
# Introduction and Technical Aspects

## Brief History and Background

Needle aspiration cytology has been in use for many decades and dates back at least to the early part of the nineteenth century. Sir James Paget is credited for aspirating malignant cells from a breast cancer patient in 1853. Much of the early experience of aspiration biopsy was not with "fine" needles but with larger bore cutting needles. The popularity of this simple procedure has largely been because of its cost effectiveness as well as the inherent qualities of the procedure itself: low complication rate, rapidity, and high diagnostic accuracy.

The incidence of breast cancer in the United States has risen, and early detection of breast cancer plays a pivotal role in prognosis and survival. Palpable lesions can be effectively biopsied using a thin needle (23 gauge or smaller) without radiologic guidance. However, with the current trend of detecting smaller, nonpalpable lesions, radiologic guidance (mostly ultrasound) is needed to adequately sample smaller lesions.

The "triple diagnostic approach," which consists of palpation, radiologic findings, and cytopathologic analysis on fine-needle aspiration (FNA), is applicable to benign, preneoplastic, borderline, and malignant diseases of the breast. Controversy continues about the use of breast FNA as the initial diagnostic modality of choice. Many issues have arisen over the past two decades that have affected the utility of this excellent procedure, including the overuse or casual application of the term *cytologic atypia* in benign breast conditions (the so-called gray zone diagnosis), which then requires tissue biopsy, and lack of understanding of the inherent limitations of the procedure by both clinicians and pathologists (such as inability to reliably distinguish in situ from invasive carcinoma). The performance and interpretation of breast FNA require adequate training and experience. Correlation with subsequent biopsies and clinical follow-up is mandatory in order to improve the diagnostic yield and accuracy of the procedure. Gray zone diagnoses as reported in the literature have ranged from 1% to 22%, with an average of 10% in most studies. Every effort should be made to minimize theses atypical/indeterminate cytologic diagnoses. However, the "gray zone" may also be the "comfort zone" for the cytopathologist, and inexperience or lack of confidence on the part of the cytopathologist may result in an increase in indeterminate diagnoses.

Overall, breast FNA is enormously successful, with an overall diagnostic sensitivity ranging from 80% to 100%, with specificity over 99%. In the modern era, breast FNA has been confronted with new roles and challenges. It is now routinely expected that breast FNA will provide an accurate diagnosis, analyze the biologic behavior of the tumor, supply biomarker information such as estrogen/progesterone receptor status, comment on cell proliferation index, and determine prognostic indicators such as Her2neu expression. These expectations can only be met if an adequate sample is obtained and the pathologist is on site to triage the material for processing.

As in other areas of diagnostic anatomic pathology, breast cytopathology has become a target for litigation. Review of the literature clearly shows that, after gynecologic cytopathology (Pap smears), breast FNA is the most common area involved in lawsuits. The most frequent problem leading to lawsuits has been overdiagnosis or false-positive diagnosis. Recently, more and more cases of underdiagnosis or false-negative reports have led to litigation partly because advancements in treatment protocols for breast cancer demonstrate that higher survival rates closely parallel early diagnosis; even short delays in diagnosis can affect prognosis. In a recent review, breast FNA accounted for 6% of all pathology-related claims (compared with breast biopsy resulting in 14% of claims). Overall, when combined (FNA, biopsy, and frozen section), almost 22% of all pathology claims are related to misdiagnoses involving breast. Overdiagnosis (rather than underdiagnosis) by either FNA or core is the most common reason, resulting in 54% of these claims. False-negative breast FNA results in that study were most commonly due to inadequate sampling. A sparsely cellular aspirate was miscalled "negative" or "fibrocystic changes." Most of these claims could have been avoided if they were initially called "nondiagnostic FNA." This is particularly important if the pathologist is not the actual aspirator and is not familiar with the clinicoradiologic findings of the case. One of the recommendations from published literature in these scenarios is to remind the clinicians (by adding a statement at the end of every FNA report) that there is a 3%–5% false-negative and a 0.5%–2% false-positive rate associated with breast FNA. Although this statement may reinforce in the clinician's mind the benefit of exercising the "triple test" strategy when dealing with a breast FNA report of these cases, most practicing pathologists (including the authors) do not believe that such a statement is routinely needed. Good communication with the radiologist or surgeon in questionable cases is more beneficial. A biopsy is strictly indicated if there is any discordance between FNA findings and the clinical or radiologic characteristics of the lesion. It is always a good idea for the pathologist to review the other two elements of this triple test (clinical and radiologic findings) and discuss them with the clinician before finalizing the report. The most common reason for a false-positive diagnosis is an interpretive error most often involving a fibroadenoma.

## Technical Aspects

Technically, breast FNA is not difficult to perform. However, the procedure requires considerable experience and should be done in conjunction with other diagnostic studies. It is widely accepted that FNA should be done and interpreted in the setting of known clinical data and mammographic studies. This is known as the *triple diagnosis* or *triple test*. When FNA is done in this setting, the need for a frozen section prior to definitive surgery is reduced. Frozen sections may still be needed, however, when the cytologic diagnosis is unsure or is at odds with the clinical data.

The current technique of FNA uses a 23- to 25-gauge needle, 1–1.5 inches long on a 10- to 20-mL syringe with or without a syringe holder. The technique can be performed with or without actual aspiration. Obtained material is smeared on slides and either alcohol fixed for Papanicolaou and hematoxylin and eosin or air dried for Romanowsky-type stains, which include Diff-Quik. Lately there has been an increase in the use of liquid-based cytology preparations in breast FNA. However, in our experience and in the experience of many others, direct smears are generally preferred to liquid-based preparations because larger cell clusters/fragments and architecture are preserved on the direct smears. It is sometimes suggested that liquid-based preparations are preferred when the operator has little experience and poor technique in the performance of FNA. We do not agree with this, as there is little a liquid-based preparation can do to make up for an inadequate sampling of a breast lesion.

Cell blocks should be prepared whenever possible. We find cell blocks superior to liquid-based preparations and direct smears for ancillary studies, and they are especially useful in estrogen receptor and progesterone receptor status determination. They also provide a reservoir of material for future studies.

On-site assessment of a fine-needle aspirate of palpable lesions is desired. Feedback to the clinician for patient management, the ability to make additional passes as needed (e.g., when lymphoma is suspected), and greater likelihood of optimal preparations are some of the benefits of immediate assessment.

Fine-needle aspiration is indicated for almost all palpable lesions to provide a rapid, accurate, and cost-effective diagnosis.

In the case of lesions such as abscesses and cysts, FNA can be a diagnostic and treatment tool. It can be used to obtain material for special studies such immunocytochemistry and molecular analysis.

The contraindications to breast FNA are almost nonexistent. The complication rate is generally quite low and the complications themselves minor. Pain, especially in the subareolar area, is reported, and rarely pneumothorax has occurred. Needle tract seeding is quite uncommon. Other more problematic complications include hemorrhage (bleeding/hematoma), infection, and vasovagal reaction. Displacement of epithelial cells or necrosis occurring during the FNA procedure can distort the aspirate or the subsequent excision and can mimic invasion of carcinoma on the final surgical excision.

Fat, stroma, and functional epithelial units containing ducts, ductules, and acini characterize the normal histology of the adult breast. A cytology specimen normally consists of fat, fibrous tissue, stromal cells, and few duct or acinar cells. These epithelial cells should be regularly shaped and arranged in honeycombed sheets. Round to oval myoepithelial cells may be present but may not be obvious (Figures 1.1 and 1.2). More glands are seen in the lactating than nonlactating female breast, and these cells have large nuclei, large nucleoli, and vacuolated cytoplasm. Breast tissue is subject to hormonal effects, such as benign secretory change. These changes, if not recognized as such, can be mistaken for atypia in breast FNA samples.

Adequacy of an aspiration is somewhat laboratory and operator dependent. If a lesion regresses after aspiration or yields only fat when a lipoma is suspected, it may be deemed adequate even if it is paucicellular. In general, more cells are required to make a benign diagnosis than a malignant one. Our laboratory uses the criteria of six clusters of epithelial cells (about 15 cells per cluster) spread over two glass slides. If the laboratory adheres to strict adequacy requirement, the number of false-negative diagnoses will decrease, but the number of unsatisfactory specimens will increase.

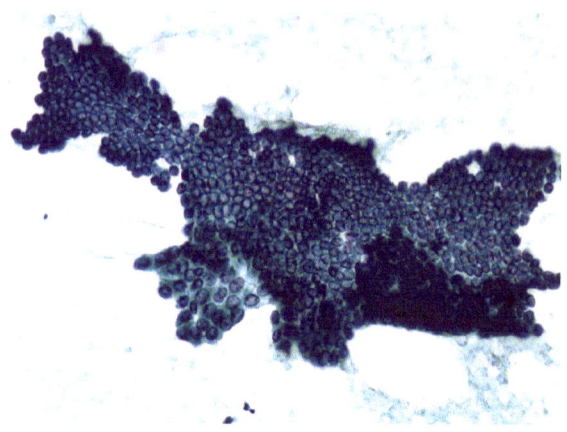

FIGURE 1.1. Normal ductal epithelium. A flat monolayered fragment of ductal epithelium with evenly spaced monomorphic nuclei. (Smear, Papanicolaou.)

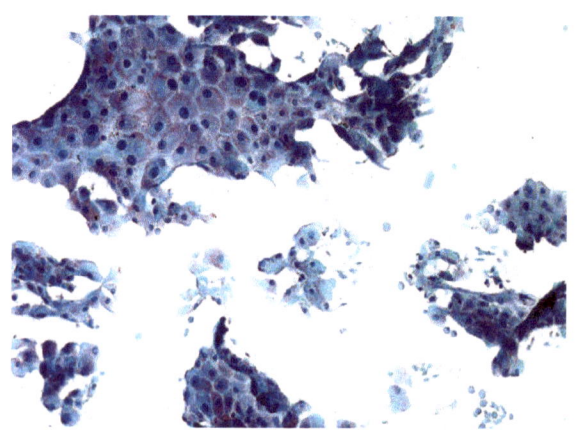

FIGURE 1.2. Metaplastic apocrine epithelium. Small fragments of large polygonal cells with abundant granular cytoplasm, each with a round nucleus with prominent nucleolus and well-defined cytoplasmic border. (Smear, Papanicolaou.)

Pitfalls in the diagnosis of breast lesions can result from poor preparation, inadequately sampled lesions, or lack of communication between the person who aspirates the lesion and the one who interprets the cytology. Some of the limitations of this procedure include the inability to distinguish in situ from invasive carcinoma, the need to evaluate further by tissue biopsy, all atypical gray zone lesions, and the lack of specific cytologic diagnoses for the majority of benign lesions.

All cytology reports should contain a statement of adequacy. This is true for the breast as well. The phrases "unsatisfactory for interpretation," "negative for malignant cells," "atypical/indeterminate," "suspicious for malignancy," and "positive for malignant cells" describe the categories often used with added statements explaining further findings.

"Unsatisfactory" is used for various reasons: poor technique, obscuring blood or inflammation, paucicellular material, and so forth. We do not encourage the use of microscopic descriptions when a specimen is unsatisfactory for interpretation. This could lead to misunderstanding on the part of the clinician reading the report. Benign is used for neoplastic as well as non-neoplastic conditions. For example: Negative for malignant cells: mastitis. Or, negative for malignant cells: fibroadenoma.

"Atypical cells present/indeterminate" indicates that the specimen is abnormal but cannot be further defined. This usually leads to additional diagnostic procedures. "Suspicious for malignant cells" is used when the suspicion of malignancy is great but perfect criteria are lacking; there may be few cells present or obscuring material. The type of malignancy suspected should be stated, that is, ductal carcinoma, sarcoma, and so forth. This category is considered positive for quality assurance and review purposes. "Positive for malignant cells" is used when malignancy is certain. Again, the type of malignancy present should be clearly stated.

## Clinical indications for breast fine-needle aspiration.

- **Diagnostic**
  - ○ Inflammatory diseases (uncommon)
  - ○ Primary neoplasms (benign vs. malignant)
  - ○ Secondary or metastatic tumors (including hematologic/lymphoid malignancies)
  - ○ Atypical epithelial lesions (require further studies)
  - ○ Tumor recurrence
- **Therapeutic**
  - ○ Evacuation of simple/inflammatory cysts

## Advantages of breast fine-needle aspiration.

- Economical/cost-effective outpatient procedure
- Minimally traumatic (physically and psychologically)
- High acceptance rate (by clinicians and patients)
- Rapid and accurate/sensitive assessment (within minutes)
- Informed pretreatment planning with the patient
- Sampling of tumor for biomarkers/molecular/ancillary studies
- Evaluation of multiple nodules/lesions
- Accurately distinguishes mastitis from inflammatory carcinoma and intramammary lymph nodes from true epithelial lesions, particularly in the area of the tail of the breast
- Avoidance of open biopsy in nonneoplastic lesions, inoperable lesions, or tumor recurrence
- May offer curative relief by cyst evacuation
- Accurate and rapid assessment of tumor recurrence in locally advanced cancer (particularly chest wall recurrence) for better tumor staging

## Major limitations of breast fine-needle aspiration.

- Inability to reliably distinguish between in situ and invasive breast carcinomas (all histologic subtypes)
- Accuracy often dependent on the size of the lesion (less sensitive below 5 mm)
- Low accuracy in tumors that are predominantly cystic/necrotic, hemorrhagic, desmoplastic, or located deep in the breast
- Lack of specific diagnosis for most benign lesions
- Need to biopsy all lesions with atypical gray zone diagnoses

## Major complications of breast fine-needle aspiration.

- Bleeding/hematoma
- Infection
- Pneumothorax
- Vasovagal reaction
- Epithelial displacement/tumor seeding
- Changes/artifacts occurring after aspiration may interfere with radiographic/ mammographic interpretation

## Major diagnostic pitfalls of breast fine-needle aspiration.

- **False-negative diagnoses**
  - Small focus of carcinoma in a background of a dominant benign lesion (such as extensive fibrocystic changes with apocrine metaplasia)
  - Carcinoma arising in a complex proliferative lesion (such as carcinoma arising in papilloma)
  - Well-differentiated carcinomas (such as in situ carcinomas, both ductal and lobular)
  - Specific histologic subtypes (such as tubular carcinoma, colloid carcinoma)
  - Rare tumor types (such as metaplastic carcinoma, apocrine carcinoma)
  - Extensively necrotic or cystic carcinoma
  - Sampling errors (in lesions that are small, deep, or have densely fibrotic stroma)
  - Poorly prepared or inadequate smears

- **False-positive diagnoses**
  - Fibroadenoma
  - Papilloma/papillary lesions
  - Atypical ductal hyperplasia
  - Pregnancy-associated or lactational changes
  - Skin adnexal tumors
  - Other lesions (such as fat necrosis, collagenous spherulosis)

## Normal cytologic constituents in breast fine-needle aspiration samples.

- Epithelium (ductal, lobular, apocrine, squamous)
- Myoepithelium
- Macrophages
- Endothelium
- Adipose, stromal, and other mesenchymal issue

*Note:* See Figures 1.1 through 1.6.

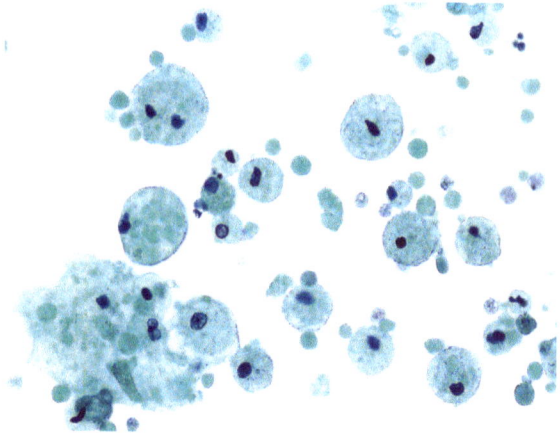

FIGURE 1.3. Foamy macrophages, breast cyst. Scattered histiocytes with abundant vacuolated cytoplasm and small uniform nuclei. Cytoplasmic border well-defined. Numerous globular structures in the background, representing cystic material. (Smear, Papanicolaou.)

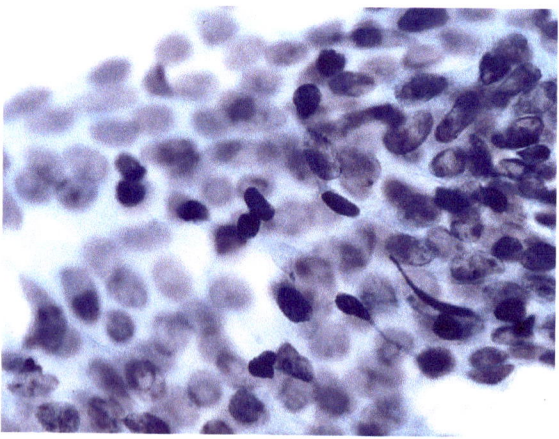

FIGURE 1.4. Myoepithelial cells. Small round to oval naked nuclei seen adherent to benign ductal epithelium. True appreciation of these cells requires focusing the cellular fragments at different planes. (Smear, Papanicolaou.)

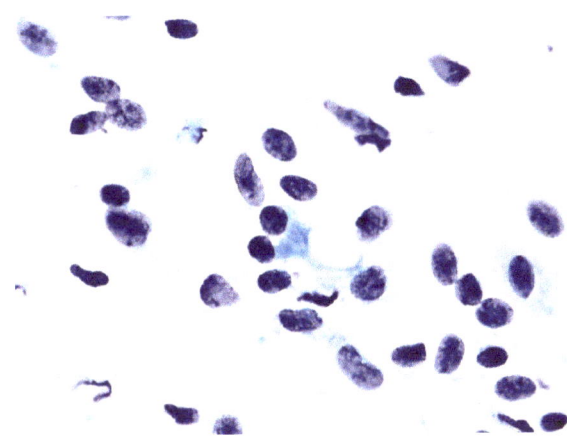

FIGURE 1.5. Myoepithelial cells. Numerous round to oval naked myoepithelial nuclei seen at higher power from a case of fibroadenoma. The presence of these cells in abundance signifies a benign lesion. (Smear, Papanicolaou.)

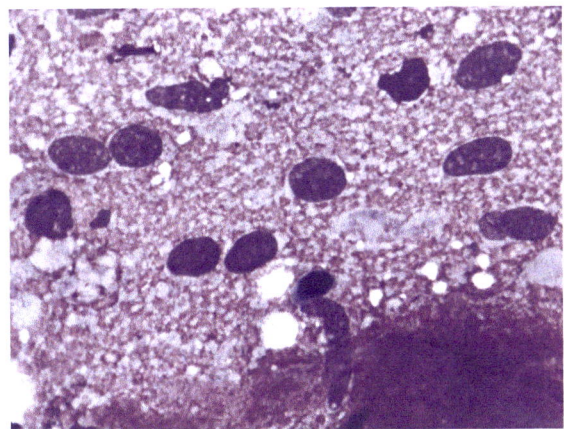

FIGURE 1.6. Myoepithelial cells. Plump, round to oval myoepithelial cell nuclei shown in a granular and vivid metachromatic background. The latter represents a stromal matrix from a fibroadenoma. (Smear, Diff-Quik.)

## Fine-needle aspiration of normal breast.

- Usually scant cellularity
- Always cohesive ductal fragments (few to no lobules)
- Uniform round nuclei, no crowding, and minimal overlap
- Dense chromatin, small inconspicuous nucleoli
- Accompanying fibroadipose tissue fragments

## Fine-needle aspiration cytologic criteria for breast carcinoma.

- Architectural characteristics (best evaluated at ×25–×40 magnification)
- Cellular morphology (best evaluated at ×100–×400 magnification)
- **General characteristics**
  - High cellularity
  - Cellular enlargement
  - High nucleus to cytoplasm ratios
  - Nuclear hyperchromasia
  - Macronucleoli (less often observed)
  - Cellular/nuclear monomorphism (not always present)
  - Eccentric nuclear placement
  - Cellular dishesion with single isolated epithelial cells
  - Mitoses/karyorrhexis
  - Cellular crowding/overlap
  - Lack of myoepithelial cells
  - Necrosis
- **Specific characteristics**
  - Small cell size with cytoplasmic lumina/vacuoles (lobular carcinoma)
  - Pleomorphic naked nuclei with macronucleoli (medullary carcinoma)
  - Abundant mucin and capillary tangles (colloid carcinoma)
  - Rigid, open-ended tubules (tubular carcinoma)

*Note:* See Figure 1.7.

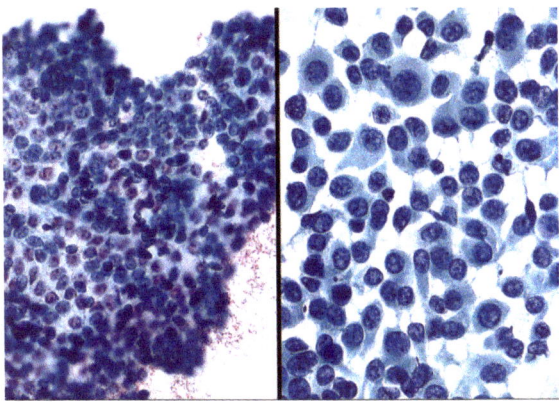

FIGURE 1.7. Cytomorphologic features comparing ductal hyperplasia **(left)** and infiltrating ductal carcinoma **(right)**. Note in ductal carcinoma the significant cellular pleomorphism, cellular dissociation, nuclear enlargement, and eccentric nuclei ("plasmacytoid" appearance). Also note the lack of myoepithelial cells. (Smear, Papanicolaou.)

Indications for fine-needle aspiration/core biopsies of palpable breast lesions.

- Palpable masses of clinical/patient concern (regardless of radiographic findings)
- Masses that can be clinically explained by normal anatomy/physiology, particularly in young patients, can be observed for two menstrual cycles
- Any persistent/suspicious masses in patients with family history should be biopsied regardless of imaging findings

*Source:* Based on data presented at the 1996 National Cancer Institute–sponsored conference.

## Indications for image-guided fine-needle aspiration/core biopsies of nonpalpable breast lesions.

- Based on the availability of high-quality breast imaging and a physician trained to interpret the findings
- Prior to image-guided biopsy, the following steps are indicated:
  ○ A complete lesion evaluation by imaging studies
  ○ A careful physical evaluation of the area of concern
- Lesions for needle core biopsies include those that are highly suggestive or suspicious for malignancy and some that have a low suspicious index but for which follow-up imaging is not feasible
- All imaging findings should be documented and procedure report made available
- Imaging results and cytopathologic/histopathologic findings should be concordant. Further work-up is needed if there is disconcordance and a follow-up recommendation made by the physician who performed the biopsies
- There should be documentation of communication among the physician performing the biopsy, the referring physician, and the patient
- All false-positive and false negative results should undergo follow-up image-guided needle biopsy

*Source:* Based on data presented at the 1996 National Cancer Institute–sponsored conference.

## Specimen adequacy for breast fine-needle aspiration (FNA).

- **Solid lesions**
  ○ No specific requirement for a minimum number of epithelial cells
  ○ Aspirator assumes the responsibility of sample adequacy based on the judgment that the FNA findings in the report are consistent with the clinical/radiographic findings
  ○ Pathologist assumes the responsibility of ensuring that the cytologic material/smears were interpretable and free from extensive artifacts
  ○ The amount of epithelial cells (few, moderate, abundant) should be reported, as well as any other cellular elements
  ○ Individual laboratories may consider specific cell count as their own criterion. There is no national standard requiring a minimal count
- **Cystic lesions**
  ○ There are no criteria for a minimal cell count. If fluid is thin, watery, and not bloody, the fluid is examined or discarded at the aspirator's discretion if the FNA completely evacuates the cyst and there is no residual palpable mass left
  ○ Any residual mass/nodule requires repeated FNA
  ○ Cysts with brown/reddish fluid (if not related to trauma of the FNA) require careful evaluation or further work-up

*Source:* Based on data presented at the 1996 National Cancer Institute–sponsored conference.

# Selected Reading

al-Kaisi N: The spectrum of the "gray zone" in breast cytology. A review of 186 cases of atypical and suspicious cytology. Acta Cytol 1994, 38:898–908.

Boerner S, Sneige N: Specimen adequacy and false-negative diagnosis rate in fine-needle aspirates of palpable breast masses. Cancer 1998, 84:344–348.

Kanhoush R, Jorda M, Gomez-Fernandez C, Wang H, Mirzabeigi M, Ghorab Z, Ganjei-Azar P: "Atypical" and "suspicious" diagnoses in breast aspiration cytology. Cancer 2004, 102:164–167.

Lee WY, Wang HH: Fine-needle aspiration is limited in the classification of benign breast diseases. Diagn Cytopathol 1998, 18:56–61.

Sidawy MK, Stoler MH, Frable WJ, Frost AR, Masood S, Miller TR, Silverberg SG, Sneige N, Wang HH: Interobserver variability in the classification of proliferative breast lesions by fine-needle aspiration: results of the Papanicolaou Society of Cytopathology Study. Diagn Cytopathol 1998, 18:150–165.

Sneige N: Fine-needle aspiration of the breast: a review of 1,995 cases with emphasis on diagnostic pitfalls. Diagn Cytopathol 1993, 9:106–112.

Tabbara SO, Frost AR, Stoler MH, Sneige N, Sidawy MK: Changing trends in breast fine-needle aspiration: results of the Papanicolaou Society of Cytopathology Survey. Diagn Cytopathol 2000, 22:126–130.

Veneti S, Daskalopoulou D, Zervoudis S, Papasotiriou E, Ioannidou-Mouzaka L: Liquid-based cytology in breast fine needle aspiration. Comparison with the conventional smear. Acta Cytol 2003, 47:188–192.

Xie HB, Salhadar A, Haara A, Gabram S, Selvaggi SM, Wojcik EM: How stereotactic core-needle biopsy affected breast fine-needle aspiration utilization: an 11-year institutional review. Diagn Cytopathol 2004, 31:106–110.

Young NA, Mody DR, Davey DD: Diagnosis and subclassification of breast carcinoma by fine-needle aspiration biopsy: results of the interlaboratory comparison program in non-gynecologic cytopathology. Arch Pathol Lab Med 2002, 126:1453–1457.

# 2
# Non-neoplastic and Proliferative Lesions

## Mastitis, Breast Abscess

In inflammatory conditions such as mastitis and abscess formation, surgery can be avoided by the use of fine-needle aspiration (FNA). In conjunction with microbiologic studies of the aspirated material, FNA can provide valuable information about the etiology of an inflammatory condition of the breast (lactation, infection, or trauma). Fine-needle aspiration can also serve as a therapeutic modality when evacuating abscess material or cyst contents.

## *Clinical Features*

- Mastitis often presents as a palpable breast lesion with varying degrees of pain and tenderness.
- Acute suppurative mastitis is typically seen in 1%–3% of lactating women in the postpartum period.
- The most common organisms are staphylococci and streptococci.
- Localized infection often results in an abscess and rarely leads to chronic mastitis with periductal inflammation, duct ectasia, fibrohistiocytic reaction, and mononuclear chronic inflammatory infiltrate.

## Cytomorphologic Characteristics

- Smear cellularity is highly dependent on the clinical stage of the lesion—high cellularity in the acute/active stage and sparse cellularity in the subacute/chronic stage due to presence of varying degrees of fibrosis.
- Smears contain abundant mixed inflammatory cells (neutrophils, lymphocytes, and plasma cells), apocrine cells, and abundant macrophages often with evidence of cytophagocytosis and multinucleated giant cells.
- Isolated cells, apocrine cells, and clusters of epithelial cells with varying degrees of reactive atypia are also present (often with an appearance reminiscent of epithelial cells in repair).

## Pitfalls and Differential Diagnosis

- Ductal carcinoma
- Fat necrosis with organized hematoma

# Chronic Subareolar Abscess

## Clinical Features

- This is considered a specific clinicopathologic entity characterized by low-grade/mild infection of the lactiferous duct or sinus leading to subsequent abscess formation and/or chronic recurrent infection and rarely fistula formation at the base of the nipple.
- Suggestion has been made that squamous metaplasia of columnar epithelial cells of the lactiferous ducts is the cause of this lesion.

## Cytomorphologic Characteristics

- High cellularity
- Mixed inflammatory infiltrate, abundance of neutrophils and lymphocytes with few plasma cells, and multinucleated giant cells

- Anucleated squamous cells, parakeratotic cells, and keratinous material
- Ductal epithelium with varying degrees of reactive atypia
- Granulation tissue
- Foamy histiocytes, cholesterol crystals

## *Pitfalls and Differential Diagnosis*

- Duct ectasia
- Ductal carcinoma with squamous differentiation, metastatic squamous cell carcinoma, and metaplastic carcinoma

## Granulomatous Mastitis

### *Clinical Features*

- Characterized by the presence of granulomatous reaction and giant cell formation
- An inflammatory lesion of either unknown etiology or the result of tuberculosis, fungal infection, epidermal inclusion cyst, or foreign body reaction such as suture and leakage from silicone implants

## *Cytomorphologic Characteristics*

- Variable cellularity (usually high)
- Epithelioid histiocytes, singly and in loose clusters
- Mixed inflammatory cells, cellular debris
- Few to abundant foreign body–type giant cells
- Ductal epithelial fragments often with significant reactive atypia

## *Pitfalls and Differential Diagnosis*

- Duct ectasia
- Low-grade ductal carcinoma

# Fibrocystic Changes

Fibrocystic changes are the most common cause of breast lumps in women between 30 and 50 years old. These are a variety of changes in the glandular and stromal tissues of the breast. Clinically, these patients may have cysts, fibrosis, tenderness, or pain. Fibrocystic breasts may make detection of breast cancer by mammography more difficult; therefore, ultrasound may be necessary in some cases if a breast abnormality is detected in a woman with fibrocystic breasts.

## *Clinical Features*

- Extremely common (50%–90% of all adult women), the most common cause of a clinically palpable breast lump
- Usually presents as a symptomatic lump with cyclical hormonal variation in size and symptomatology
- Young to middle aged women, peak incidence just before menopause
- Usually bilateral and multifocal
- May mimic breast cancer clinically, radiologically, and cytopathologically
- Causation not exactly known, perhaps hormonal (excess of estrogen, low progesterone, or their imbalance)
- Primarily affects the terminal duct lobular unit
- Characterized by presence of gross and microscopic cysts, apocrine metaplasia, and blunt duct adenosis
- May be accompanied by epithelial proliferation of varying degrees, which should be reported separately

## *Cytomorphologic Characteristics*
(Figures 2.1 to 2.3)

- Smears usually hypercellular with a varying admixture of different cell types, including apocrine cells
- Usually cohesive fragments of ductal epithelium—"honeycomb fragments," often with focal to confluent apocrine

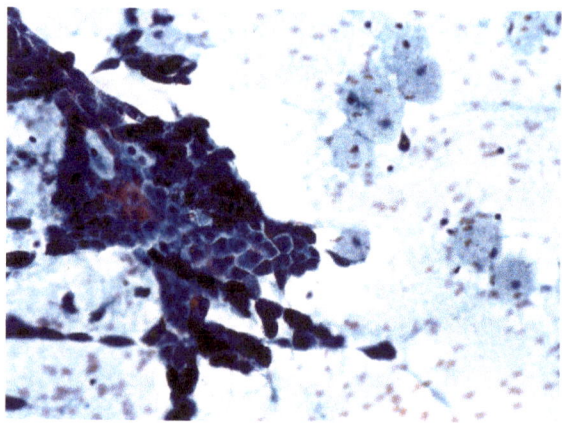

FIGURE 2.1. Fibrocystic changes. A partially folded fragment of apocrine cells seen in a background of numerous foamy macrophages and cystic debris. (Smear, Papanicolaou.)

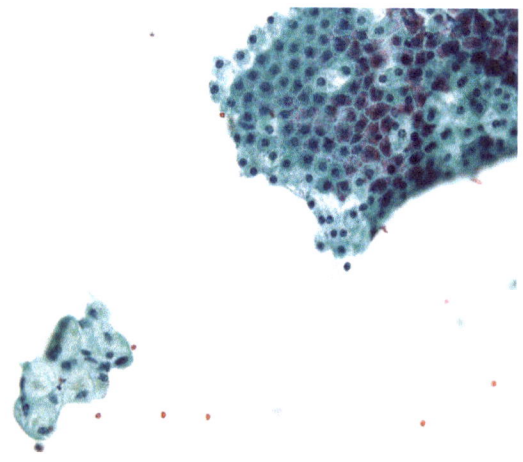

FIGURE 2.2. Fibrocystic changes. A flat monolayered fragment of apocrine epithelium alongside a cluster of large foamy macrophages. (Smear, Papanicolaou.)

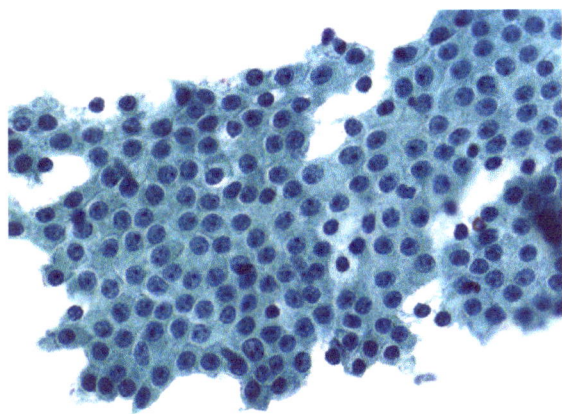

FIGURE 2.3. Fibrocystic changes. A large fragment of apocrine cells arranged in a large monolayered fashion. Cells are large and polygonal with large nuclei and prominent nucleoli with abundant granular cytoplasm. Apocrine epithelium is a fairly common finding in breast aspirates and, except for rare occasions, represents benign lesions. (Smear, Papanicolaou.)

metaplasia (large polygonal cells, abundant cytoplasm that is distinctly granular, well-defined cytoplasmic borders, often prominent nucleoli)
- Mild anisonucleosis, slight nuclear overlap
- Sometimes macrophages predominate, often with foamy cytoplasm—"foamy macrophages"
- Myoepithelial cells, fragments of stroma, adipose tissue
- Background of cystic debris
- Rarely, microcalcifications (calcified debris)

## Pitfalls and Differential Diagnosis
- Atypical ductal hyperplasia
- Fibroadenoma
- Low-grade ductal carcinoma

# Proliferative Breast Disease

Proliferative changes in the breast may be associated with an increased risk for breast cancer. This category is composed of epithelial hyperplasia, with or without atypia. The interobserve variability for the interpretation of this group of breast lesions (particularly when associated with atypia) is extremely high with poor cytohistologic correlation.

## Clinical Features

- Mild ductal hyperplasia, adenosis, cystic changes, and apocrine metaplasia are not associated with an increased risk of cancer.
- Peripheral breast disease without atypia is associated with a slightly higher risk (1.5–2.0 times) of breast carcinoma.
- Examples of peripheral breast disease without atypia include sclerosing adenosis, moderate to florid epithelial hyperplasia, and papillomatosis.
- These lesions may be seen with or without accompanying fibrocystic changes or some other benign breast lesion.
- Peripheral breast disease with atypia, including atypical ductal hyperplasia and atypical lobular hyperplasia, are clinically significant lesions with a much higher risk for subsequent development of breast cancer (four to five times).

## Cytomorphologic Characteristics
(Figures 2.4 to 2.7)

- There is moderate to high cellularity.
- Tightly cohesive ductal epithelial fragments are abundant.
- The degree of epithelial proliferation can be subdivided into mild, florid, and atypical.
- Dual cell population (epithelial/myoepithelial) is present in peripheral breast disease but only focally and minimally noted in atypical ductal hyperplasia.

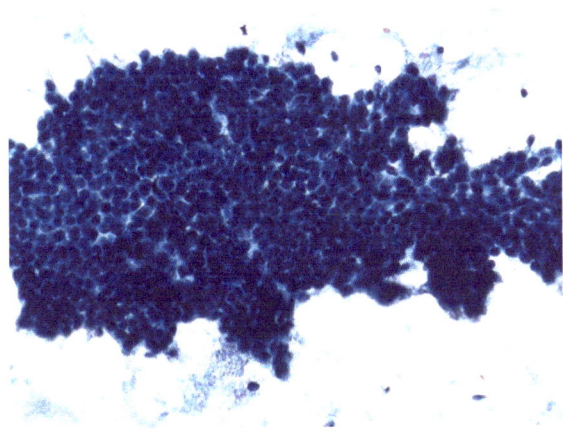

FIGURE 2.4. Usual ductal hyperplasia. A large fragment of ductal epithelium with mildly enlarged and crowded nuclei. Note the cohesive nature of the fragment and relative preservation of the flat, honeycombed architecture. A closer inspection would also reveal myoepithelial nuclei. (Smear, Papanicolaou.)

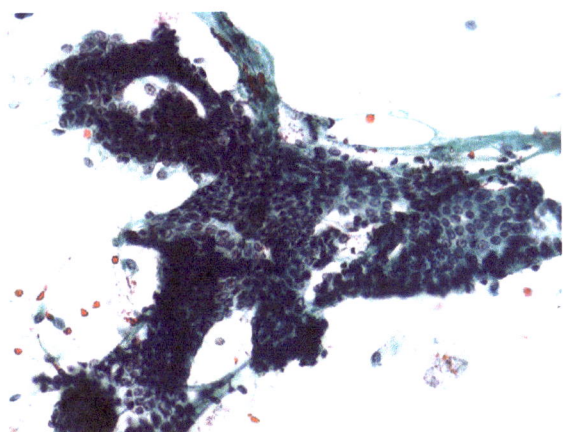

FIGURE 2.5. Atypical ductal hyperplasia. Breast epithelium displaying a more complex architecture with branching and sharply punched out spaces. Cells have enlarged and hyperchromatic nuclei. Myoepithelial cells are often appreciated in these fragments. Note the cohesive nature of the cellular fragments and the lack of individually dispersed epithelial cells in the background, a feature often seen in ductal carcinoma. (Smear, Papanicolaou.)

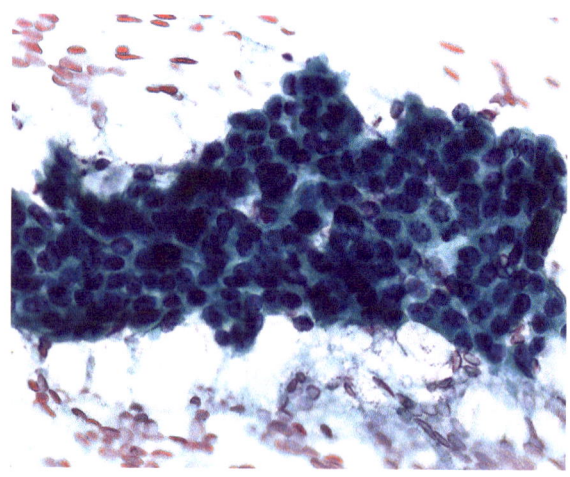

FIGURE 2.6. Atypical ductal hyperplasia. At higher magnification, this case illustrates markedly enlarged and hyperchromatic nuclei imparting a crowded look to the cellular fragment. The fragment still depicts a cohesive architecture with lack of individually dispersed epithelial cells. Although the cytologic features are worrisome, the follow-up revealed multifocal atypical ductal hyperplasia. (Smear, Papanicolaou.)

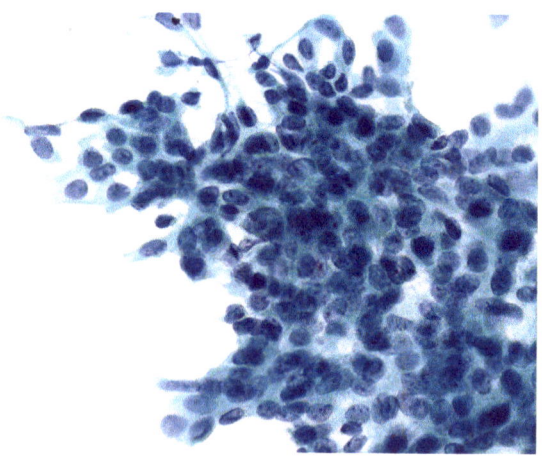

FIGURE 2.7. Atypical ductal hyperplasia. Cellular fragment displaying more pleomorphism with enlarged crowded nuclei and the beginning of a three-dimensional architecture. The cells are loosely cohesive at the fragment edges. (Smear, Papanicolaou.)

- Some associated features of fibrocystic changes may be present in peripheral breast disease but rarely in atypical ductal hyperplasia.
- Predominantly moderately crowded cellular fragments with minimal pleomorphism, lack of cellular dissociation, or single cells (peripheral breast disease). Atypical ductal hyperplasia may show a much greater degree of cellular crowding and nuclear overlap, with a varying but small number of atypical loosely cohesive cells (see Figures 2.6 and 2.7).
- Occasional papillary or, more often, pseudopapillary configurations are present.
- Cytologic atypia (lack of polarity/organization, nuclear enlargement and overlap, micronucleoli) is present in atypical ductal hyperplasia.
- Cribriformlike architecture, three-dimensional epithelial fragments with slitlike spaces/lumens, and complex infoldings of epithelial fragments are noted in atypical ductal hyperplasia.
- Myoepithelial nuclei are usually identified, often in different planes of focus in peripheral breast disease. *Florid atypical ductal hyperplasia may lack myoepithelial cells.*
- Lobular hyperplasia is characterized by an increase in the amount of intact lobular units, often with clearly visible small lumens and minimal cellular crowding. In atypical lobular hyperplasia the lumens get smaller with appreciable cellular crowding and disorganization of the epithelium.

## Pitfalls and Differential Diagnosis

- Low-grade ductal carcinoma. Presence of cytologic monomorphism, high cellularity, and single cells favor ductal carcinoma
- Fibroadenoma
- Papilloma

## Fine-needle aspiration reporting in peripheral breast disease.

- Proliferative breast disease (no clinical recommendation)
- Proliferative breast disease with mild atypia (recommendation: clinical follow-up)
- Proliferative breast disease with florid/severe atypia (recommendation: tissue biopsy)

It is imperative to render the above interpretations in the context of the "triple test" in order to avoid a false-positive cancer diagnosis.

## Cytomorphologic comparison between atypical ductal hyperplasia and ductal carcinoma in situ on fine-needle aspiration.

- The cytomorphologic distinction between atypical ductal hyperplasia and low-grade invasive ductal carcinoma in situ is often difficult and may not always be possible to make.
- Studies have shown that, in general, cases of atypical ductal hyperplasia are most likely to be diagnosed as negative or atypical. In contrast, ductal carcinoma in situ is more likely to be interpreted as suspicious or positive.
- Features favoring atypical ductal hyperplasia include sheetlike architecture, flat or monolayered and cohesive cells, finely granular chromatin, distinct cell borders, and presence of myoepithelial nuclei.
- Features favoring ductal carcinoma in situ include more single dishesive atypical cells, loosely arranged epithelial fragments, prominent anisonucleosis, coarser nuclear chromatin ("clumped chromatin"), and background inflammatory cells.
- Other cellular characteristics (nuclear size, nucleus to cytoplasm ratios, hyperchromasia, macronucleoli) show a significant overlap and are not helpful.

# The Issue of Gray Zone Cytopathology

Sometimes breast FNA cannot render an unequivocal diagnosis of a benign lesion or carcinoma. Studies have shown that the gray zone diagnoses may represent 7%–20% of all breast FNAs and are often a cause of frustration for both the cytopathologist and the clinician.

## Common Reasons for Gray Zone Diagnoses

- Technical (usually the most common culprit)
  - Sparse cellularity
  - Obscuring blood, air-drying artifact

If it is unsatisfactory for evaluation, state this in the diagnosis. Do not attempt to interpret as "atypical" if the smears cannot be evaluated due to the above factors, or, worse, do not commit to a positive diagnosis.

- Interpretative, pathologist-related: lack of experience in breast FNA. The gray zone diagnosis is like a comfort zone for the interpreter. Inexperience leads to a larger comfort zone where the interpreter would not want to be definitive in his or her diagnosis. The influence of adequate training and experience cannot be overemphasized in breast cytopathology.
- Interpretative, overlapping cytomorphologic features or "true gray zone": significant and real morphologic overlap exists between atypical/benign and atypical/malignant lesions.

## Common Sources of Gray Zone Diagnoses

Benign

- Fibroadenoma (the common and the most "notorious" cause)
- Intraductal papilloma
- Atypical ductal hyperplasia
- Gynecomastia

Malignant

- Intracystic papillary carcinoma
- Infiltrating lobular carcinoma
- Apocrine carcinoma
- Tubular carcinoma

*Published Accounts and Authors' Experiences of Practical Problems in Gray Zone Diagnoses*

- Cellular fibroadenoma versus ductal carcinoma
- Solitary ductal papilloma versus intracystic papillary carcinoma
- Apocrine metaplasia versus well-differentiated apocrine carcinoma
- Lobular carcinoma versus benign breast lesions (lactational changes)
- Tubular carcinoma versus benign breast (or fibroadenoma)
- Atypical ductal hyperplasia versus cribriform ductal carcinoma in situ

# Columnar Cell Lesions of the Breast

Columnar cell lesions are increasingly encountered in breast FNA in women between the ages of 35 and 50 years. It can be a common finding in breasts with microcalcifications or can be an incidental finding in fibroadenomas or fibrocystic changes. These peculiar lesions involve the terminal duct lobular unit and display well-formed columnar cells with apical secretory snouts, also called CAPSS or "columnar alteration with prominent apical snouts and secretions." Columnar cell lesions represent a spectrum of proliferative epithelial change with and without significant cytologic atypia. These are often nonpalpable lesions that could be multifocal or bilateral in the breasts. Most common histologic follow-up finding is benign fibrocystic change. The clinical significance of columnar cell lesions is not well-defined; however, they can be seen in association with lobular lesions (atypia, in situ carcinoma) and tubular carcinoma.

When FNAs are performed on these lesions, the most common scenario is a palpable breast mass or a radiographic density or nodule. Cytomorphologically, moderate to abundant three-dimensional cellular fragments are seen composed of polygonal round to oval cells. There is usually a loss of polarity especially toward the center of the fragments where cellular crowding and disorganization are quite pronounced. Characteristically, the cells at the periphery display columnar morphology with prominent palisading in the long axis. Rarely flat sheets with branchings and infoldings are also seen. Secretory snouts are seen in up to half of the cases on FNA. Myoepithelial cells are almost always present intermingled with the ductal epithelium. Some cases have a significant number of single epithelial cells requiring a careful evaluation to avoid overdiagnosis, as significant atypia is rarely seen in such cells. Foamy histiocytes and apocrine metaplastic cells are rare.

Differential diagnosis of columnar cell lesions includes papilloma, fibroadenoma, low-grade ductal carcinomas, and postradiation changes.

# Silicone Mastitis

## *Clinical Features*

- Often associated with ruptured silicone tissue expanders
- Exuberant proliferative tissue reaction may result in single or multiple nodules simulating malignancy

## *Cytomorphologic Characteristics*
(Figures 2.8 to 2.11)

- Characterized by pools or globs of liquid silicone, often surrounded by epithelioid histiocytes, foamy macrophages, or foreign body–type giant cells forming "silicone granulomata"
- Cytohistologic picture may also resemble fat necrosis
- Smears are moderately cellular

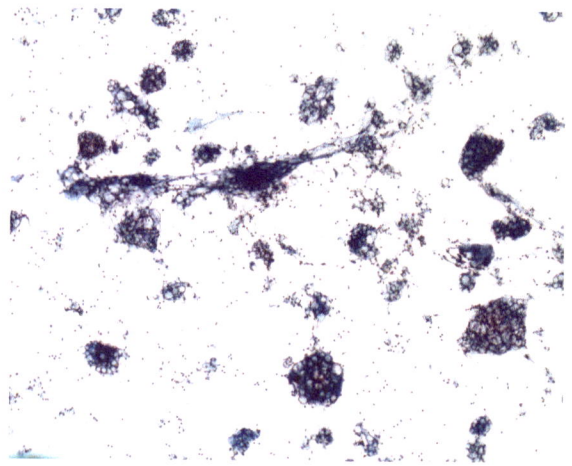

FIGURE 2.8. Silicone mastitis. A hypercellular smear displaying numerous irregular fragments of markedly distended histiocytes resembling adipose tissue fragments. Numerous inflammatory cells seen in the background. (Smear, Papanicolaou.)

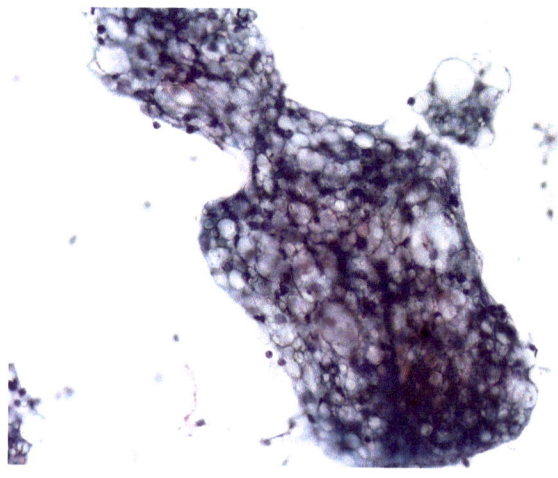

FIGURE 2.9. Silicone mastitis. A large cluster of tightly packed histiocytes. The cytoplasm appears clear and is markedly distended due to the presence of silicone material. (Smear, Papanicolaou.)

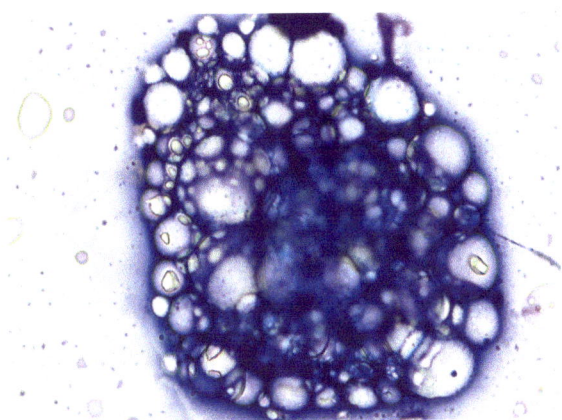

FIGURE 2.10. Silicone mastitis. Higher magnification reveals pale yellow refractile silicone material within the cytoplasm of the histiocytes. (Smear, Diff-Quik.)

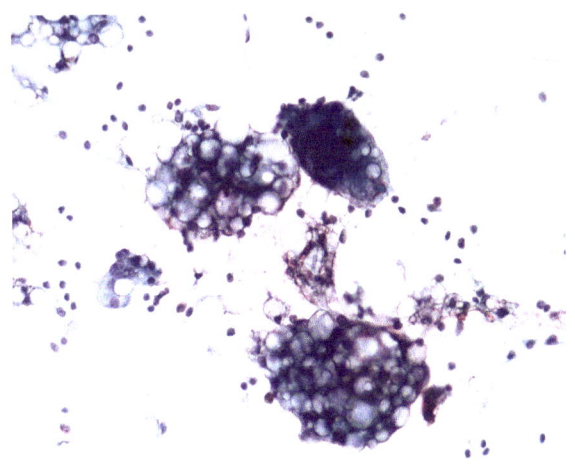

FIGURE 2.11. Silicone mastitis. Several clusters of silicone-containing histiocytes, multinucleated giant cells, and background lymphocytes representing a granulomatous reaction. (Smear, Papanicolaou.)

- Aggregates of distended macrophages, with refractile cytoplasmic globules
- Inflammatory cells, multinucleated giant cells
- Degenerated, often vacuolated, adipocytes

## *Pitfalls and Differential Diagnosis*

- Fat necrosis
- Ductal carcinoma
- Lipoma

## Fat Necrosis/Organizing Hematoma

### *Clinical Features*

- Trauma-induced inflammatory conditions
- History of trauma may or may not be available
- Mammographically, fat necrosis with subsequent calcification may also mimic a neoplastic process
- May result in a firm, irregular, fixed, and painful breast mass
- Mimics breast cancer not only clinically and radiologically but also cytopathologically
- May create diagnostic problems if the history of injury is remote or is not recalled by the patient

### *Cytomorphologic Characteristics*
(Figures 2.12 to 2.17)

- Scant cellularity (rarely smears appear hypercellular due to abundance of inflammatory cells, histiocytes, and endothelial proliferation)
- Abundant foamy or hemosiderin-containing macrophages, lymphocytes, plasma cells, fibroblasts, and fragments of fibrous tissue and newly formed vessels
- Degenerated/necrotic fat cells/vacuoles, often with calcified debris and dirty granular background, lipophages
- Occasional multinucleated foreign body–type giant cells

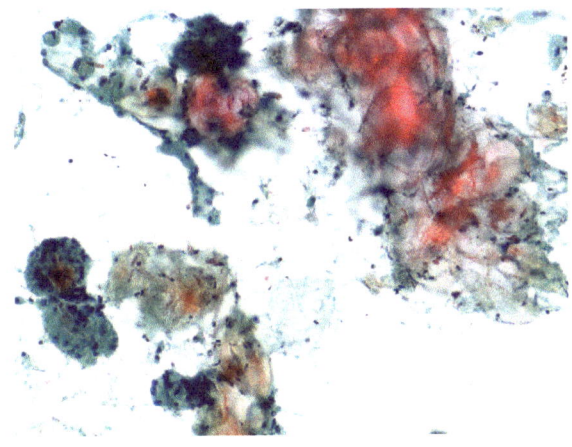

FIGURE 2.12. Fat necrosis. Degenerated fat, histiocytes, and multinucleated foreign body–type giant cells. (Smear, Papanicolaou.)

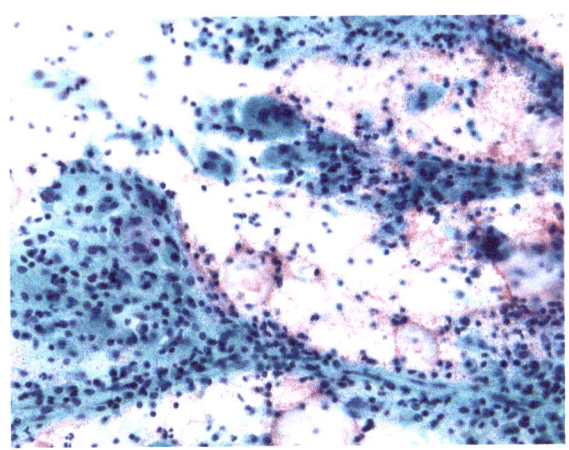

FIGURE 2.13. Fat necrosis. Hypercellular smear depicting degenerated fat, chronic inflammatory cells, and multinucleated histiocytes. Abundant fine capillary vessels represent formation of granulation tissue. (Smear, Papanicolaou.)

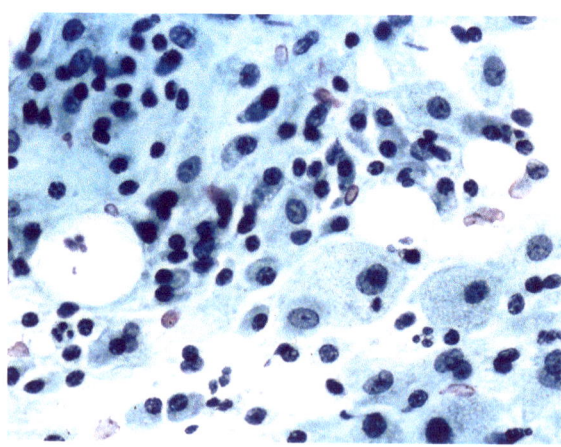

FIGURE 2.14. Fat necrosis. Higher magnification illustrating the polymorphous composition of the cellular infiltrate, that is, lymphocytes, plasma cells, endothelial cells, and foamy macrophages. (Smear, Papanicolaou.)

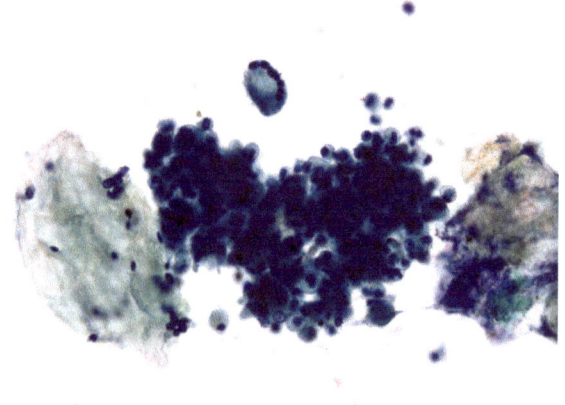

FIGURE 2.15. Fat necrosis. Higher magnification illustrates degenerated fat, a tight aggregation of inflammatory cells, and histiocytes and multinucleated giant cells. (Smear, Papanicolaou.)

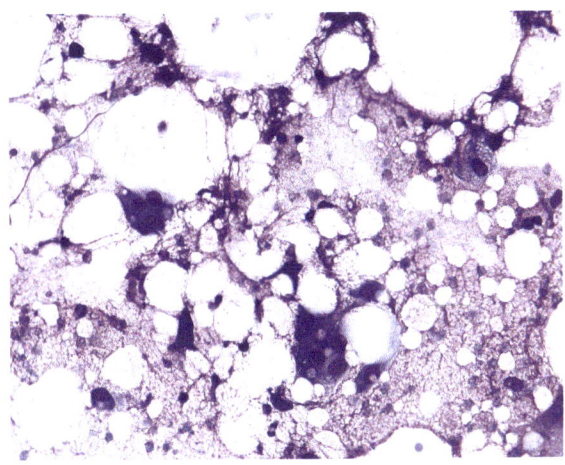

FIGURE 2.16. Fat necrosis. High magnification shows small clusters of histiocytes embedded within a degenerated, granular background. Caution should be taken not to overcall these cells as infiltrating carcinoma cells. (Smear, Diff-Quik.)

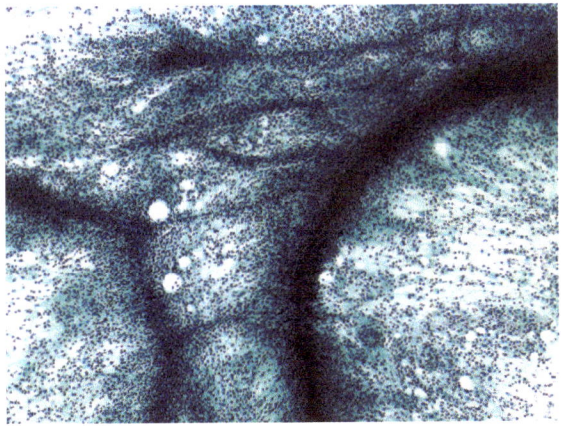

FIGURE 2.17. Fat necrosis with organizing hematoma. Hypercellular smear composed of inflammatory cells, histiocytes, and proliferating endothelial cells, which is a common accompaniment of granulation tissue formation. (Smear, Papanicolaou.)

- "Chicken-wire" or arborizing capillaries, often with proliferating fibroblasts
- Epithelioid histiocytes can be overinterpreted as malignant epithelial cells; and/or ductal epithelial fragments present in the smear are overcalled because of the significant reactive atypia present
- Reactive epithelial atypia associated with fat necrosis has resulted in false-positive diagnoses of cancer

## Pitfalls and Differential Diagnosis

- Ductal carcinoma

## Mucocelelike Lesion

### Clinical Features

- Rare lesion often quite small, usually a diagnostic problem on FNA (differentiation from mucinous carcinoma)
- Often associated with fibrocystic changes and is thought to originate from ruptured mucinous cyst into breast stromal tissues

## Cytomorphologic Characteristics
(Figures 2.18 and 2.19)

- Smears with scant cellularity
- Small epithelial fragments, monomorphic, lack of atypia
- Abundant background mucin
- Muciphages, in varying numbers
- Occasional bare myoepithelial nuclei

## Pitfalls and Differential Diagnosis

- Colloid carcinoma

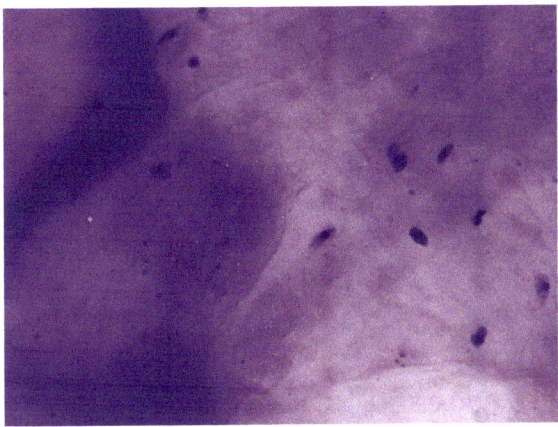

FIGURE 2.18. Mucocele. Thick, abundant mucinous background containing rare macrophages. These lesions are devoid of ductal epithelium, a helpful finding to distinguish them from well-differentiated mucinous carcinoma. (Smear, Diff-Quik.)

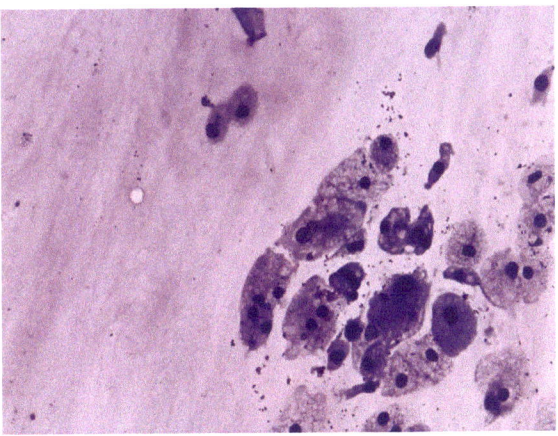

FIGURE 2.19. Mucocele. Higher magnification shows numerous mucin-containing macrophages in a thick mucinous background. (Smear, Diff Quik.)

# Radiation-Induced Changes

## *Clinical Features*

- Radiation-induced changes are not uncommon because a larger proportion of patients are undergoing breast-conserving therapies that may include adjuvant radiation.
- The effects of radiation are noted not only in any residual carcinoma but also in the nonneoplastic mammary tissue.

## *Cytomorphologic Characteristics* (Figure 2.20)

- Smears usually paucicellular
- Small epithelial fragments, often lobular in nature, with significant cytologic atypia (vacuolated cytoplasm, enlarged nuclei, prominent nucleoli) and degenerative changes

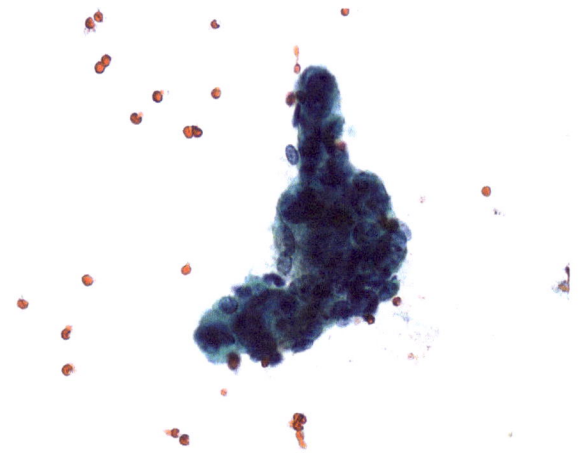

FIGURE 2.20. Radiation atypia. Partially intact breast lobule with markedly enlarged, pleomorphic nuclei displaying macronucleoli. The patient had a history of radiation treatment for ductal carcinoma. Although the morphologic changes are too bizarre to represent lobular carcinoma, such cases require a careful interpretation when patients have previously resected breast cancer. (Smear, Papanicolaou.)

- Lymphomononuclear inflammatory cells
- Rarely fat necrosis (in cases of recent surgery/biopsy)
- If significant atypia, can lead to erroneous false-positive diagnosis of cancer on aspiration

## *Pitfalls and Differential Diagnosis*

- Atypical lobular hyperplasia
- Ductal or lobular carcinoma

## Collagenous Spherulosis

Collagenous spherulosis is an uncommon lesion, first described in 1987, characterized by the presence of distinct globules of amorphous material that resemble adenoid cystic carcinoma histologically and cytologically.

## *Clinical Features*

- Usually an incidental microscopic finding, often accompanying benign proliferative lesions of the breast such as sclerosing adenosis, radial scar, and intraductal papilloma
- Can be unifocal or multifocal

## *Cytomorphologic Characteristics*
(Figures 2.21 to 2.25)

- Smears are moderately cellular with monolayered fragments of epithelium, often with a focal branching papillary architecture
- Metachromatic "hyaline" globules (on Diff-Quik stain), pale green and vaguely translucent (on Papanicolaou stain), usually well formed, surrounded by monomorphic ductal epithelial cells
- Higher magnification reveals fibrillar structures of the globules, which often vary in size

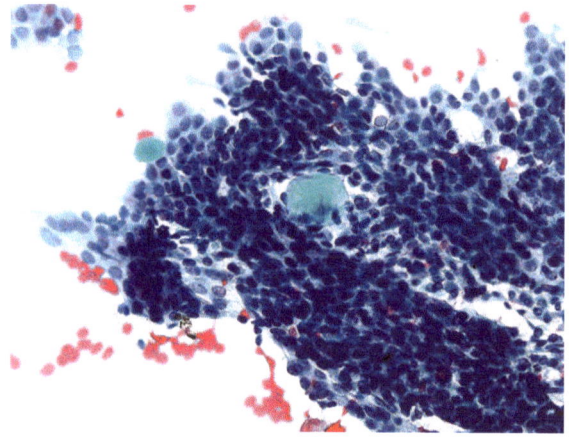

FIGURE 2.21. Collagenous spherulosis. Cellular smear with hyper-chromatic and crowded ductal epithelium. Two well-defined pale green globular structures are present. (Smear, Papanicolaou.)

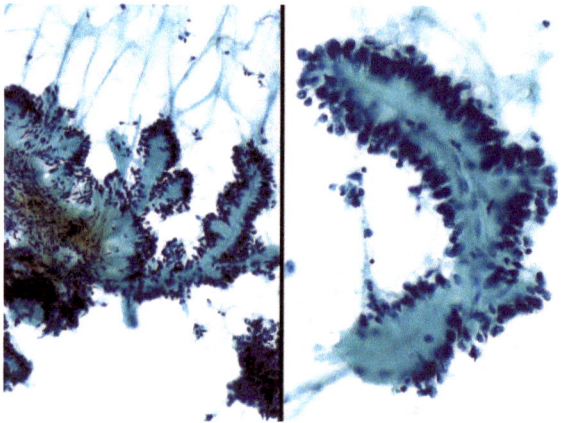

FIGURE 2.22. Collagenous spherulosis. Papillary-like branching cords of pale green cylindrical structures lined by proliferative ductal epithelium. Note the presence of stromal nuclei within the pale green substance, a feature often helpful in distinguishing collagenous spherulosis from adenoid cystic carcinoma. (Smear, Papanicolaou.)

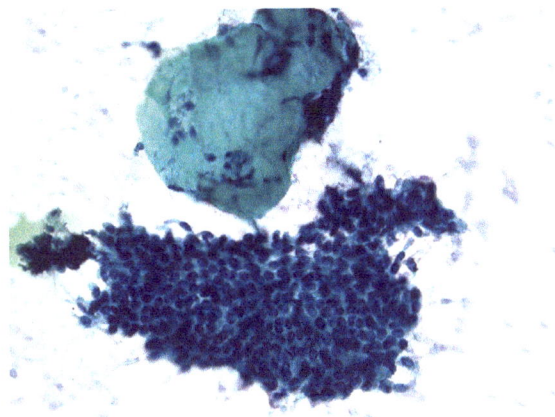

FIGURE 2.23. Collagenous spherulosis. High magnification of a hyperchromatic crowded ductal epithelial fragment and juxtaposed pale green sharply defined globular structure. A morphologic distinction from adenoid cystic carcinoma can be extremely difficult. (Smear, Papanicolaou.)

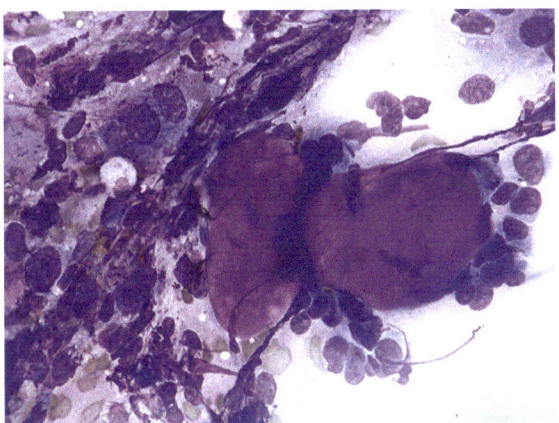

FIGURE 2.24. Collagenous spherulosis. Higher magnification of metachromatic spherules mimicking adenoid cystic carcinoma. The presence of loosely cohesive ductal epithelial cells in the background makes it an extremely treacherous cytomorphologic interpretation. The presence of other associated findings in the case (such as papillomatosis and sclerosing adenosis) are often helpful for the diagnosis of collagenous spherulosis. (Smear, Diff-Quik.)

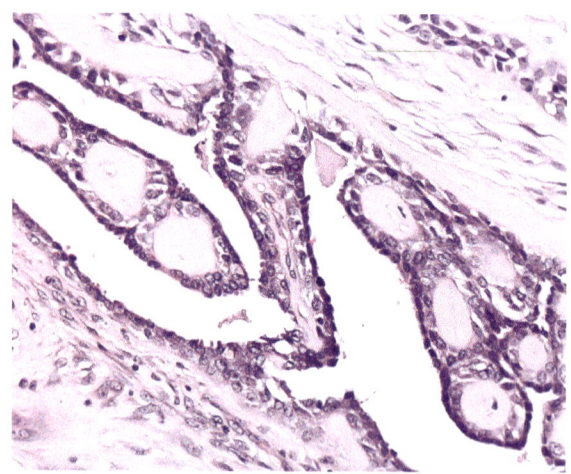

FIGURE 2.25. Collagenous spherulosis. Histologic section illustrating at high magnification the source of the amorphous globular structures seen in a fine-needle aspiration smear of this entity. Note the presence of well-defined myoepithelial cells surrounding these pale eosinophilic structures. (Histologic section, hematoxylin and eosin.)

- Lack of significant cellular atypia, lack of basaloid nature of the accompanying epithelium
- Occasional papillary ductal epithelial fragments or associated changes of a benign papilloma
- Diagnostic confusion with adenoid cystic carcinoma may lead to a false-positive diagnosis of cancer on FNA

## Pitfalls and Differential Diagnosis

- Adenoid cystic carcinoma
- Ductal carcinoma in situ, cribriform type
- Adenomyoepithelioma, tubular variant

# Pregnancy/Lactational Changes and Lactational Adenoma

## *Clinical Features*

- These changes and adenomas are uncommonly encountered.
- Fine-needle aspiration distinction between lactational change and lactating adenoma is difficult (if at all possible).
- The lesions may lead to an erroneous false-positive diagnosis of carcinoma because of the atypical cytologic features. A careful clinical history of pregnancy/lactation should always be sought when rendering a diagnosis of carcinoma in a younger patient.

## *Cytomorphologic Characteristics*
(Figures 2.26 to 2.30)

- Hypercellular smears, "yielding" FNAs
- Loosely cohesive ductal or, more often, lobular epithelial fragments
- More intact lobular fragments in lactating adenoma, often with prominent secretory changes (cytoplasmic vacuoles); prominent outer myoepithelial cell layer
- Usually larger cells, with prominent nucleoli and foamy cytoplasm; cytoplasm is extremely fragile and wispy
- Numerous round, naked nuclei in the background (epithelial cell nuclei), often with prominent nucleoli
- Numerous inflammatory cells (mostly mature polymorphous lymphocytes), few macrophages
- Proteinaceous and frothy slide background, often hemorrhagic, obscuring cellular details

## *Pitfalls and Differential Diagnosis*

- Galactocele
- Fibroadenoma, tubular adenoma
- Atypical ductal hyperplasia, atypical lobular hyperplasia

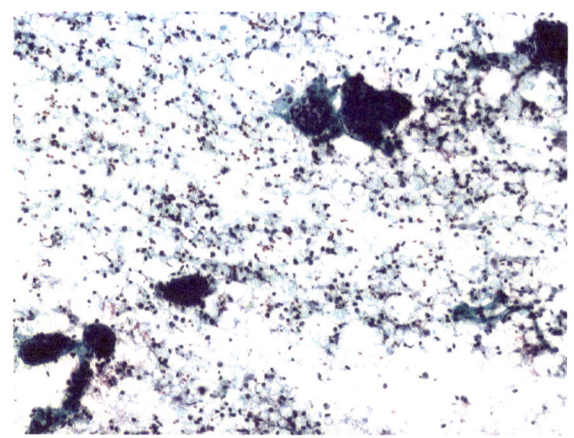

FIGURE 2.26. Lactational change. Hypercellular smear composed of distended breast lobules and abundant mixed inflammatory cells in the background. These findings may appear worrisome leading to an erroneous diagnosis of atypia or cancer. (Smear, Papanicolaou.)

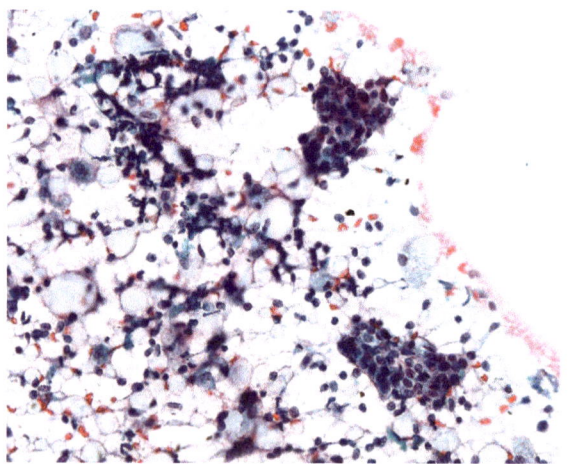

FIGURE 2.27. Lactational change. Hypercellular smear that at higher magnification reveals partially disrupted lobules with enlarged hyperchromatic nuclei. Numerous naked lobular cell nuclei are present in the background in addition to lymphocytes, histiocytes, and numerous large lipid vacuoles. (Smear, Papanicolaou.)

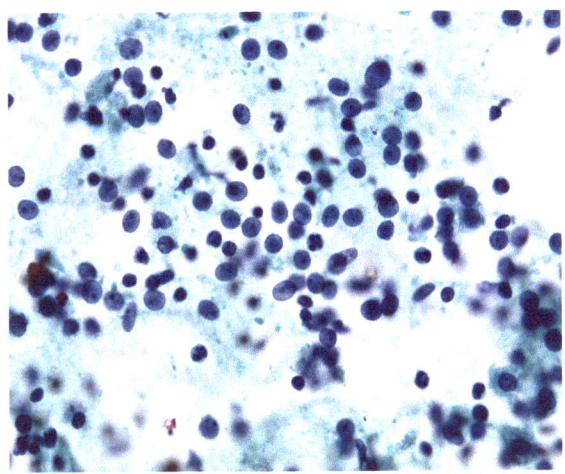

FIGURE 2.28. Lactational change. A totally dissociated population of naked nuclei of lobular cells admixed with mixed inflammatory cells is present. The presence of prominent nucleoli is unusual for lobular carcinoma. The observer should have a much higher threshold for interpreting atypia or cancer when dealing with a fine-needle aspirate from a young pregnant or lactating patient. (Smear, Papanicolaou.)

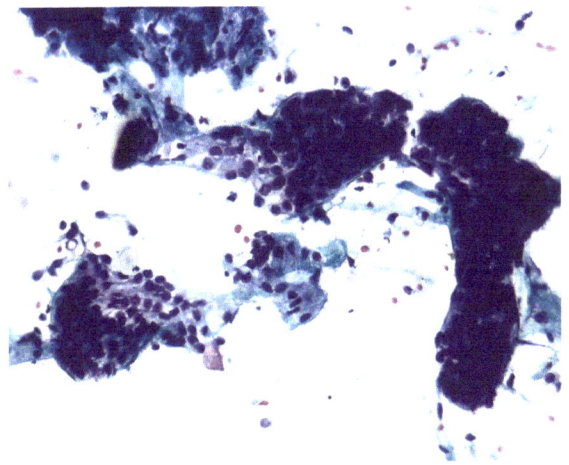

FIGURE 2.29. Lactational change. Intact breast lobules distended with enlarged and hyperchromatic epithelial cells. Note the well-defined myoepithelial cell layer around these lobular structures. A casual look at such aspirates may result in a false-positive diagnosis of lobular carcinoma. (Smear, Papanicolaou.)

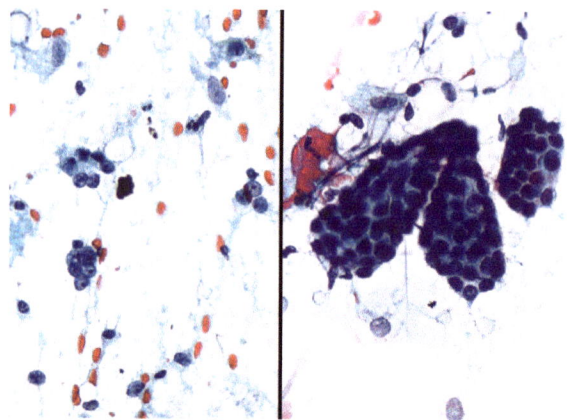

FIGURE 2.30. Lactational change. Higher magnification in the left panel illustrates cytologically atypical, dispersed lobular cells appearing as naked nuclei with prominent nucleoli. The background is granular and shows occasional lipid vacuoles. Distinction from lobular carcinoma would be extremely difficult in such cases. The case on the right shows similar cells, but they are in more intact lobules. (Smear, Papanicolaou.)

- Ductal or, more often, lobular carcinoma
- Non-Hodgkin lymphoma

## Gynecomastia

Male breast masses are uncommon pathologic findings. They are rarely aspirated, resulting in limited cytopathologic experience (male breast FNAs account for 1.4%–7.3% of all breast FNAs). However, male breast FNA is considered to be a highly sensitive (95.3%) and specific (100%) diagnostic procedure. Gynecomastia is defined as male breast enlargement caused by both hypertrophy and hyperplasia of the ductal epithelial and stromal components. Although the etiologic factors may vary, the condition is essentially caused by a relative increase in estrogenic activity, a decrease in androgenic activity, or a combination of both.

## Clinical Features

- Usually located in the subareolar region
- Presents clinically as a unilateral or bilateral, tender, and often painful mass, which has a flat "discoid" appearance on palpation
- Bimodal age distribution (adolescents and adults, often in the sixth decade)
- Higher incidence recently observed in human immunodeficiency virus–positive patients receiving antiretroviral therapy

## Cytomorphologic Characteristics
(Figures 2.31 to 2.34)

- Variable cellularity, most often moderate (however, cellularity can often be low because of the fibrous nature of the lesion, and the discomfort that the patient experiences at the time of aspiration is due to an often extreme tenderness)
- Large cohesive ductal epithelial fragments, often papillary-like or flat and monolayered; often a prominent cribriform architecture is seen
- Focal to confluent epithelial atypia, sometimes quite significant with cellular crowding, nuclear enlargement, and prominent nucleoli
- Small amount of scattered background myoepithelial nuclei
- Atypical single epithelial cells rarely observed (useful feature when distinguishing gynecomastia from a male breast ductal carcinoma)
- Occasional fragments of metachromatic stromal/fibrous tissue (may appear falsely biphasic resembling a fibroadenoma)

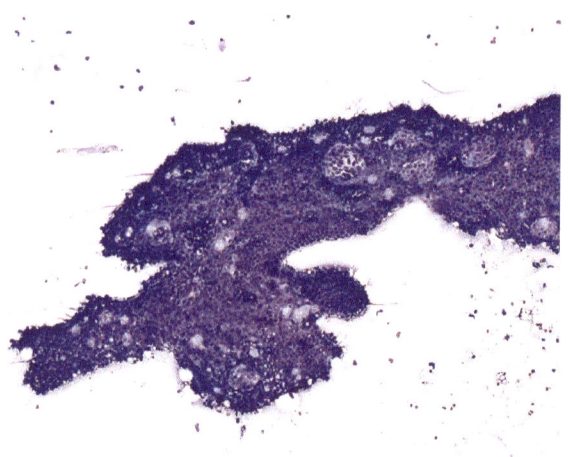

FIGURE 2.31. Gynecomastia. A large fragment of hyperplastic ductal epithelium with a vague papillary and cribriform architecture is seen. Note the presence of numerous naked myoepithelial cells in the background. (Smear, Papanicolaou.)

FIGURE 2.32. Gynecomastia. A biphasic architecture composed of cohesive hyperplastic ductal epithelium and myxoid stroma. Numerous myoepithelial cells are seen in the background. (Smear, Diff-Quik.)

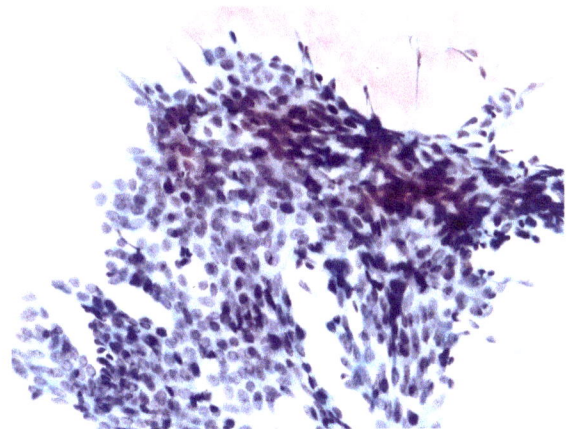

FIGURE 2.33. Gynecomastia. An atypical ductal epithelial fragment with large crowded nuclei. A total lack of individually dispersed epithelial cells helps to rule out carcinoma in these cases. (Smear, Papanicolaou.)

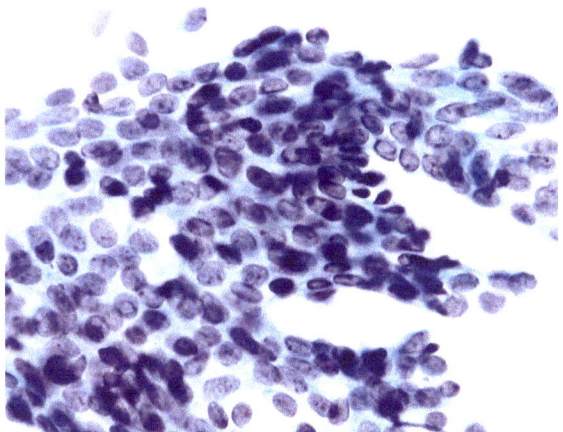

FIGURE 2.34. Gynecomastia. Higher magnification of a ductal epithelial fragment shows enlarged crowded nuclei with occasional myoepithelial cells. One should have a much higher threshold for an atypical/cancer diagnosis in a male breast aspiration because of the significant cytologic atypia in these lesions and the rarity of male breast carcinoma. (Smear, Papanicolaou.)

## *Pitfalls and Differential Diagnosis*

- Ductal carcinoma
- Atypical ductal hyperplasia
- Metastatic tumors (most commonly, lung adenocarcinoma)
- Fibroadenoma (This possibility is uncommonly raised because of the often biphasic appearance in gynecomastia. The usual source of the loose metachromatic material often seen in Diff-Quik–stained smears of gynecomastia is the myxomatous change often noted in the periductular location of these lesions.)
- Male breast carcinoma (Because carcinoma of male breast is exceedingly rare, it should always be ruled out first; this is particularly critical because gynecomastia can harbor significant epithelial atypia. One should have a much higher threshold for a cancer diagnosis when dealing with male breast aspirates. Male breast carcinoma, which is almost always the ductal type, shows greater pleomorphism, smaller tissue fragments, more single cells, and total lack of myoepithelial cell nuclei [Figures 2.35 and 2.36].)

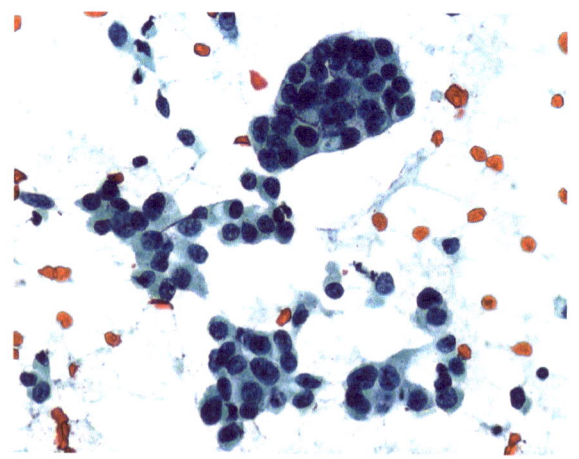

FIGURE 2.35. Ductal carcinoma in male breast. (Smear, Papanicolaou.)

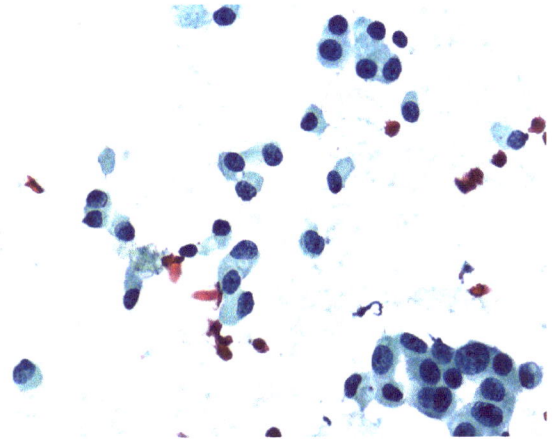

FIGURE 2.36. Ductal carcinoma in male breast. Higher magnification of the view in Figure 2.35 illustrates enlarged, pleomorphic, hyperchromatic nuclei that are eccentrically placed in the cytoplasm, imparting a plasmacytoid appearance. (Smear, Papanicolaou.)

# Inflammatory Myofibroblastic Tumor

Inflammatory myofibroblastic tumor is an uncommon benign tumorlike lesion that rarely occurs in the breast. The lesion in the breast resembles its more common lung counterpart. Fine-needle aspiration experience with inflammatory myofibroblastic tumor in the breast is extremely limited.

## Clinical Features

- Inflammatory myofibroblastic tumor has been observed in most human organs.
- Clinically and on radiographic studies, it may simulate a primary breast carcinoma.
- There are no systemic or constitutional symptoms of infection noted.
- This is a rare lesion with many synonyms: inflammatory pseudotumor, plasma cell granuloma, inflammatory myofibroblastic tumor, fibroxanthoma, and so forth.

- A small subset show molecular/chromosomal evidence of a neoplastic nature. However, most lesions are thought to be related to infectious etiology.
- Immunoexpression of the ALK protein as a result of chromosomal translocation involving 2p23 is seen in a number of cases.

## Cytomorphologic Characteristics

- A proliferative process of myofibroblasts
- Sparsely cellular aspirates
- Characterized by benign cellular features with a polymorphous population of mostly chronic inflammatory cells, plus histiocytes and spindled fibroblasts (or myofibroblasts)
- Benign-appearing ductal epithelium may be present, as well as connective tissue fragments
- Some features may resemble fat necrosis
- Vascular-endothelial proliferation often noted
- Histiocytes and spindled cells may show well-formed intranuclear inclusions
- No granulomas

## Pitfalls and Differential Diagnosis

- Granulomatous mastitis
- Fat necrosis
- Granular cell tumor
- Fibromatosis
- Metaplastic carcinoma
- Myofibroblastoma

# Primary Amyloid Tumor

## Clinical Features

- Primary amyloid tumors are rare nonneoplastic lesions.
- Clinically and radiologically, the findings are often indeterminate, necessitating FNA.

- Breast can be involved as an isolated organ-specific manifestation or as part of systemic amyloidosis.
- Patients often do not have clinical or pathologic evidence of amyloidosis, monoclonal gammopathy, or plasma cell dyscrasias.

## Cytomorphologic Characteristics

- Sparsely cellular
- Aggregates of birefringent, dense irregular amorphous material of varying sizes, some with embedded nuclei of lymphomononuclear cells
- The waxy hyaline nature is highlighted on Papanicolaou stain when it assumes a pale green/blue hue
- Numerous background lymphocytes
- Occasional multinucleated giant cells
- Congo red reactivity with apple green birefringence is diagnostic

## Pitfalls and Differential Diagnosis

- Adenoid cystic carcinoma
- Chondroid syringoma

# Pseudoangiomatous Stromal Hyperplasia

Pseudoangiomatous stromal hyperplasia is a benign fibroblastic or myofibroblastic stromal lesion with well-described histologic phenotype characterized by the formation of numerous anastomosing slitlike spaces in an often densely hyalinized stroma. It shares a superficial resemblance to low-grade vascular tumor, hence the name *pseudoangiomatous*.

## Clinical Features

- Pseudoangiomatous stromal hyperplasia may present as a well-defined noncalcified and homogeneous nodular mass or, more commonly, coexist with other breast lesions (gynecomastia, hamartoma, etc.).

- Some cases are proven to be hormonally related.
- This hyperplasia is more common in premenopausal women and postmenopausal women receiving hormone replacement therapy. Some cases show size fluctuations during menses.
- Myofibroblasts in pseudoangiomatous stromal hyperplasia immunoexpress hormone receptors (particularly progesterone).
- This hyperplasia grows slowly. Rarely has rapid growth been reported in immunocompromised patients.
- Local excision is curative in most cases.
- Its exact nature is unclear; it could be related to an underlying neoplastic process, as some cases recur locally after excision.

## Cytomorphologic Characteristics

- Aspirates are often extremely scant and mostly nondiagnostic (because of stromal hyalinization).
- When diagnostic, the smears are scantly cellular and display cohesive benign-appearing ductal fragments, often in flat sheets, less often as branching structures, "fibroadenomalike"
- Rare, bland-appearing spindled cells
- Numerous single bipolar naked nuclei
- Bipolar uniform spindled cells
- Hypocellular loose stromal tissue fragments or fibrillary matrix
- No cellular pleomorphism, no mitoses

## Pitfalls and Differential Diagnosis

- Fibroadenoma
- Phyllodes tumor
- Myofibroblastoma
- Metaplastic carcinoma

# Reactive Spindle Cell Nodules

Reactive spindle cell nodules are uncommon, benign, non-neoplastic lesions that arise following FNA procedures. The needle trauma to certain breast lesions incites a localized myofibroblastic proliferation suggesting an exuberant reactive response as a cause for reactive spindle cell nodules.

## *Clinical Features*

- Most present as unencapsulated tiny nodules measuring up to 10 mm in size.
- Interestingly, most reactive spindle cell nodules are seen in association with papillary and complex sclerosing breast lesions.

## *Cytomorphologic Characteristics*

- Morphologically, the lesions in the breast are similar to those seen in thyroid, salivary glands, and urinary bladder.
- Smears show spindled cells with mild pleomorphism.
- Fine arborizing capillary vessels are present.
- Inflammatory cells and macrophages are present.
- Immunoexpression of smooth muscle markers is diagnostically helpful.

## *Pitfalls and Differential Diagnosis*

- Myofibroblastoma
- Pseudoangiomatous stromal hyperplasia
- Metaplastic carcinoma

## *Selected Reading*

Allen EA, Parwani AV, Siddiqui MT, Clark DP, Ali SZ.: Cytopathologic findings in breast masses in men with HIV infection. Acta Cytol 2003, 47:183–187.

Bardales RH, Stanley MW: Benign spindle and inflammatory lesions of the breast: diagnosis by fine-needle aspiration. Diagn Cytopathol 1995, 12:126–130.

Dodd LG, Sneige N, Reece GP, Fornage B: Fine-needle aspiration cytology of silicone granulomas in the augmented breast. Diagn Cytopathol 1993, 9:498–502.

Filomena CA, Jordan AG, Ehya H: Needle aspiration cytology of the irradiated breast. Diagn Cytopathol 1992, 8:327–332.

Jain S, Gupta S, Kumar N, Sodhani P: Extracellular hyaline material in association with other cytologic features in aspirates from collagenous spherulosis and adenoid cystic carcinoma of the breast. Acta Cytol 2003, 47:381–386.

Jain S, Kumar N, Sodhani P, Gupta S: Cytology of collagenous spherulosis of the breast: a diagnostic dilemma—report of three cases. Cytopathology 2002, 13:116–120.

Kumarasinghe MP: Cytology of granulomatous mastitis. Acta Cytol 1997, 41:727–730.

Siddiqui MT, Zakowski MF, Ashfaq R, Ali SZ: Breast masses in males: multi-institutional experience on fine-needle aspiration. Diagn Cytopathol 2002, 26:87–91.

Silverman JF, Lannin DR, Unverferth M, Norris HT: Fine needle aspiration cytology of subareolar abscess of the breast. Spectrum of cytomorphologic findings and potential diagnostic pitfalls. Acta Cytol 1986, 30:413–419.

# 3
# Benign and Borderline Tumors

## Fibroadenoma

Fibroadenoma is the most common benign tumor occurring in the breast of adolescent and young women, typically noted between the ages of 20 and 35 years. It is rare before puberty and in the postmenopausal period and may show increased growth during pregnancy and lactation.

### *Clinical Features*

- A fibroadenoma is usually a solitary, firm, discrete, well-circumscribed nodule (usually 2–3 cm), freely mobile in the breast.
- There can be multiple lesions in the ipsilateral or even in the contralateral breast.
- It is a fibroepithelial tumor with a characteristic biphasic appearance.
- It may be confused clinically or radiologically with breast cyst or an intramammary lymph node.
- Rarely carcinomas have been reported in fibroadenomas (usually in situ or invasive lobular carcinoma).

## Cytomorphologic Characteristics
(Figures 3.1 to 3.8)

- Grossly, the aspirate may appear sticky and tenacious, often clogging the needle lumen.
- Smears are often hypercellular with a characteristic biphasic appearance (epithelium and mesenchymal/stromal tissue).
- Epithelium appears as cohesive, usually monolayered sheets of well-organized ductal-type epithelium, often with foldings, branchings with a "papillarylike" architecture ("staghorn") or even tubular.
- Naked bipolar myoepithelial nuclei are noted scattered in the smear background in a significant number of cases. These have the so-called rice grain morphology and are best visualized in Papanicolaou-stained smears.
- Variably cellular fibrous stromal fragments are present.
- Chondromyxoid stroma is present, often with a bright metachromatic or magenta-colored appearance on Diff-Quik–stained smears and less obvious on Papanicolaou-stained smears (pale green).
- Juvenile fibroadenomas tend to have a more monomorphic appearance with predominantly larger epithelial fragments of a blander uniform columnar type. A papillary architecture can be a prominent feature.
- Uncommon features include significant epithelial atypia (nuclear enlargement, crowding, pleomorphism, and prominent nucleoli), apocrine and foam cells, prominent mucinous change, multinucleated giant cells, and lack of a stromal component (see Figures 3.5 to 3.8).

## Pitfalls and Differential Diagnosis

- Fibrocystic changes
- Atypical ductal hyperplasia
- Intraductal papilloma, papillary carcinoma
- Pyllodes tumor

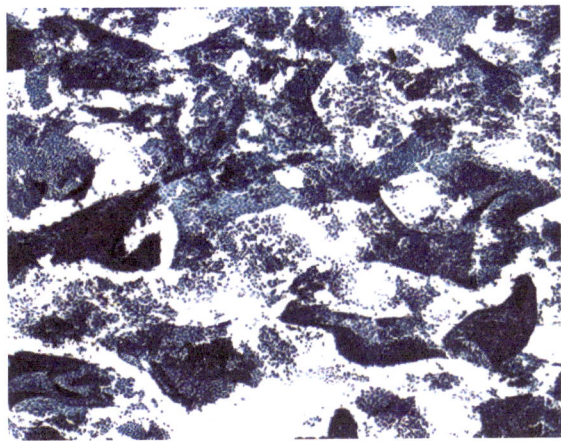

Figure 3.1. Fibroadenoma. The case illustrates the degree of hyper-cellularity that can be encountered in these tumors. There are numerous branching fragments of ductal epithelium admixed with background myoepithelium. (Smear, Papanicolaou.)

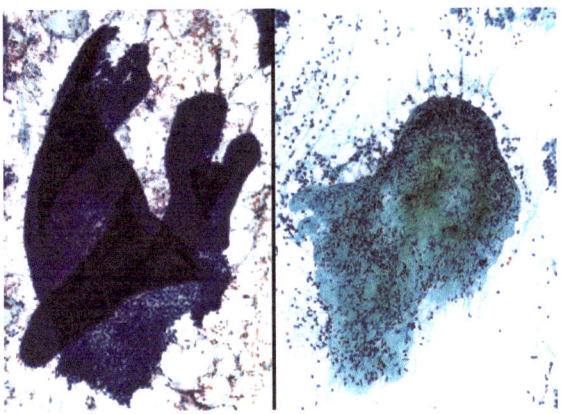

Figure 3.2. Fibroadenoma. A branching ductal epithelial fragment with the characteristic staghorn appearance is shown on the left. A combination of stromal matrix with mesenchymal cell proliferation and abundant myoepithelial cells is observed on the right. (Smear, Papanicolaou.)

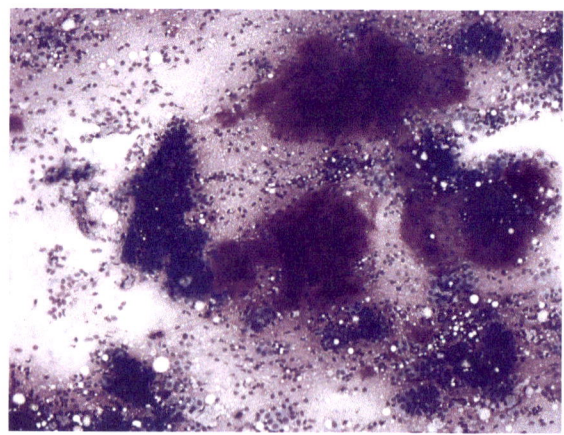

FIGURE 3.3. Fibroadenoma. Hypercellular smear displaying biphasic morphology of the tumor. The smear shows ductal epithelial fragments, bright magenta-colored stromal matrix containing fusiform mesenchymal cell nuclei, and abundant background naked myoepithelial cell nuclei. (Smear, Diff-Quik.)

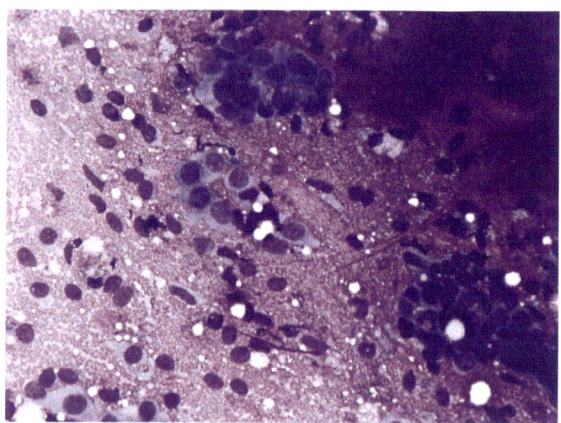

FIGURE 3.4. Fibroadenoma. High magnification shows ductal epithelium with enlarged crowded nuclei, granular-appearing magenta stromal matrix, and naked myoepithelial cell nuclei. (Smear, Diff-Quik.)

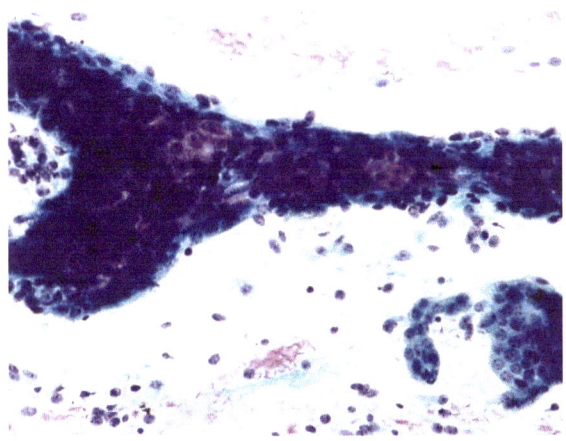

FIGURE 3.5. Fibroadenoma. This branching tubular structure can be confused with a well-differentiated tubular carcinoma. However, the presence of numerous background myoepithelial nuclei is extremely helpful to exclude malignancies. (Smear, Papanicolaou.)

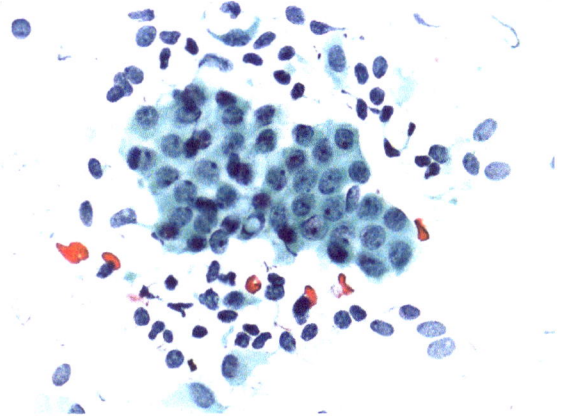

FIGURE 3.6. Fibroadenoma. A higher magnification shows cytologic atypia of the ductal epithelium with enlarged nuclei and occasional prominent nucleoli. Numerous myoepithelial cell nuclei are present in the background. The diagnosis of fibroadenoma is typically rendered on an appreciation of the cellular architecture at lower magnifications. A significant degree of cytologic atypia is often present in these tumors and can lead to diagnostic confusion when an aspirate of fibroadenoma is evaluated at higher magnifications. (Smear, Papanicolaou.)

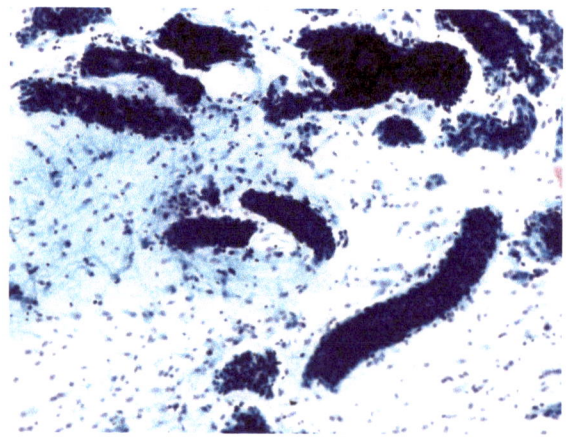

FIGURE 3.7. Fibroadenoma. Numerous well-defined tubules of atypical ductal epithelium mimic tubular carcinoma. However, the presence of abundant myoepithelium is extremely helpful in accurately diagnosing this lesion as benign. (Smear, Papanicolaou.)

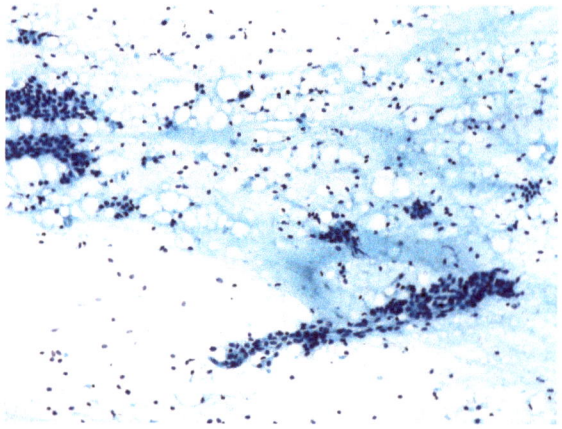

FIGURE 3.8. Fibroadenoma. The presence of abundant mucin is an uncommon finding in this tumor and may create diagnostic confusion with colloid carcinoma. However, the lack of overt malignant epithelial characteristics and the presence of abundant myoepithelial cells exclude carcinoma. In these cases the source of mucin is thought to be either epithelial mucin from dilated glandular lumens or mucinous change of the stromal matrix. (Smear, Papanicolaou.)

- Low-grade ductal carcinoma (particularly tubular carcinoma)
- Mucinous carcinoma

# Phyllodes Tumor

A phyllodes tumor is a rare fibroepithelial breast tumor often distinguished from fibroadenoma by the presence of a more prominent and cellular mesenchymal component. It is a major differential diagnosis of a breast lesion with a significant spindle cell or mesenchymal component. Although most phyllodes tumors are benign, low-grade (borderline) and malignant subtypes are occasionally encountered. Their preoperative distinction from fibroadenomas (which is not always possible) is considered clinically significant, as phyllodes tumors are resected with a wider negative margin in order to avoid tumor recurrence.

## *Clinical Features*

- Occurrence is rare, accounting for 0.3%–1% of primary breast tumors.
- Peak incidence is seen much later in life than fibroadenoma (45–50 years).
- Most patients present with a unilateral slowly enlarging breast mass, with an average size of 5 cm.
- Approximately 15%–20% of phyllodes tumors recur after excision.

## *Cytomorphologic Characteristics*
(Figures 3.9 to 3.13)

- Hypercellular smears, biphasic but more often epithelial-predominant (in benign tumors), with large stromal fragments ("phyllodes fragments"), often in an anatomizing/branching pattern

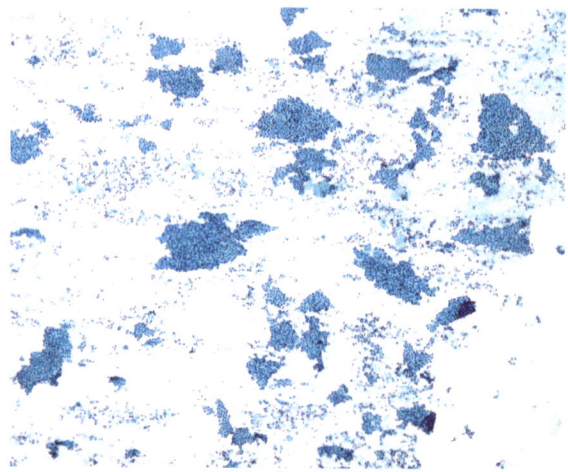

FIGURE 3.9. Benign phyllodes tumor. Hypercellular smear composed of large, irregular fragments of ductal epithelium, loose myxoid/mucinous stroma, and abundant myoepithelium. A cytomorphologic distinction from fibroadenoma would be extremely difficult. (Smear, Papanicolaou.)

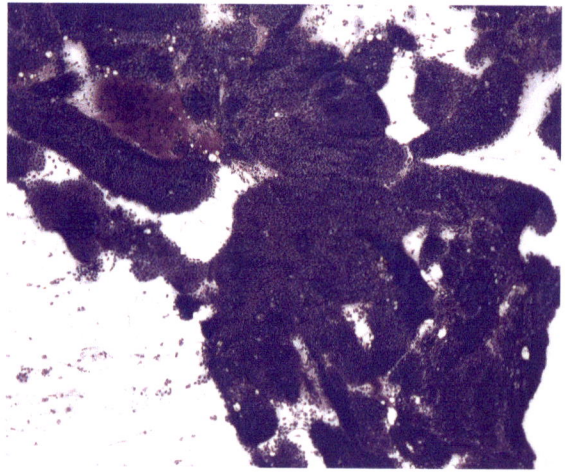

FIGURE 3.10. Benign phyllodes tumor. Hypercellular smear consists predominantly of irregular branching ductal epithelium. A small amount of myxoid stroma is noted at 11:00 o'clock. (Smear, Diff-Quik.)

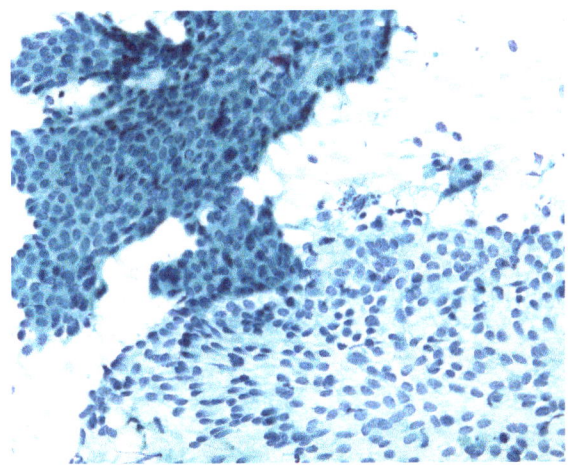

FIGURE 3.11. Benign phyllodes tumor. High magnification shows the classic biphasic morphology. The ductal epithelial fragment shows enlarged, somewhat crowded nuclei, whereas the stromal component shows round to oval and fusiform nuclei embedded in a loose myxoid tissue. (Smear, Papanicolaou.)

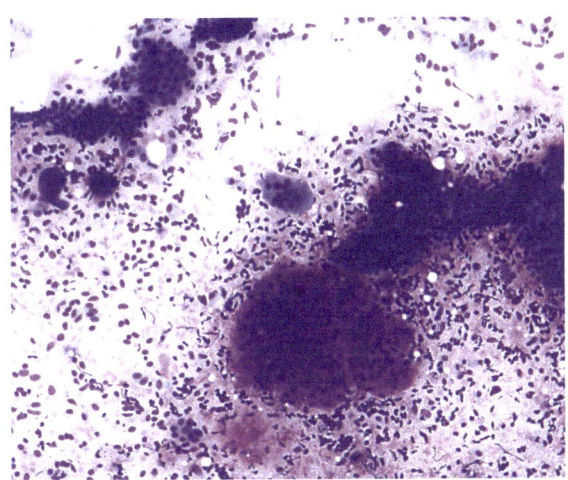

FIGURE 3.12. Benign phyllodes tumor. Hypercellular smear shows crowded fragments of ductal epithelium, stromal matrix, myoepithelial cells, multinucleated giant cells, and numerous individually dispersed mesenchymal cell nuclei. (Smear, Diff-Quik.)

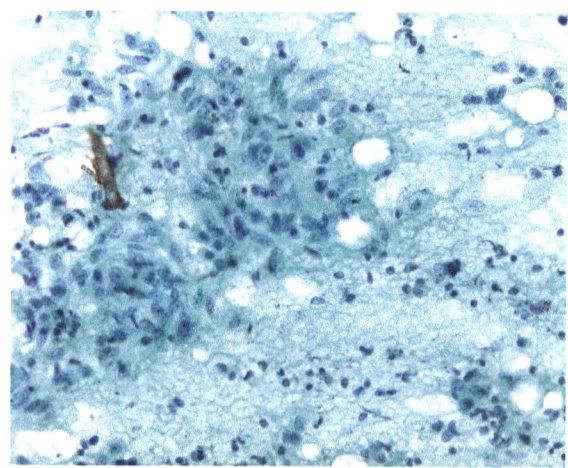

FIGURE 3.13. Benign phyllodes tumor. Higher magnification of these stromal components shows pleomorphic fusiform nuclei and numerous myoepithelial cell nuclei. (Smear, Papanicolaou.)

- Large, often folded, bland-appearing cohesive epithelial fragments
- Dissociated spindle and stromal/mesenchymal cells (seen more often in the malignant tumors) with plump fusiform nuclei often associated with myxoid or mucinous stromal tissue (metachromatic on Diff-Quik stain)
- Rarely, chondroid metaplasia
- Occasional mitotic figures in the stromal cells
- Stromal fragments most often with monomorphic cells, but occasional significant atypia (pleomorphic spindle cells)
- Occasional multinucleated giant cells, apocrine ductal cells, or foam cells
- Malignant phyllodes tumor is significantly more hypercellular, depicting more stromal predominance and more atypia of the dissociated stromal cells (The stromal cells may appear fibrosarcomalike or stromal sarcomalike in these cases. Positive immunostaining with p53 in this scenario remains a contentious issue.)

## Pitfalls and Differential Diagnosis

- The distinction between fibroadenoma and phyllodes tumor in an aspirate is based on the cellularity of the stromal elements seen in phyllodes tumors and is not always possible to visually appreciate. The size of the lesion is not a valid distinguishing feature.
- Diagnosis of low-grade or malignant phyllodes tumor is extremely difficult. These cases should be carefully evaluated for the presence of abnormal mitoses and pleomorphism. Other entities that may be considered in the differential diagnosis include fibromatoses and certain sarcomas.
- Occasionally phyllodes tumors can be deceptively hypocellular, lacking the characteristic stromal fragments. This may happen if the needle samples the focally hyalinized or myxoid areas of the tumor. Therefore, adequate sampling of the lesion should always be attempted by multiple aspirations.

## Intraductal Papilloma/Papillomatosis

Papilloma is a benign tumor of ductal origin, most often seen in larger subareolar lactiferous ducts. It is most often solitary, although multiple tumors can be seen in the peripheral breast. Bilateral tumors are rare. Intraductal hyperplasia with papillary architecture or "papillomatosis" is a nonspecific entity denoting a phenotypic appearance, which should be distinguished from a true intraductal papilloma. Less often, papilloma comes to attention as a mass lesion (may measure up to 3 cm) in the fifth to sixth decades of life (somewhat younger than for patients with papillary carcinoma).

## Clinical Features

- Usually presents with nipple discharge, often serous or blood-tinged

- Less often visualized on routine mammograms as a small mass or a dilated duct; occasionally have microcalcifications
- Mostly in older women; may be seen in young children or men
- Multiple papillomas often associated with concurrent atypical duct hyperplasia or ductal carcinoma in situ
- Uneventful outcome in most cases, with only 6% recurrence rate following excision (Approximately 6% of the patients develop carcinomas, with majority of them having invasive disease.)

## Cytomorphologic Characteristics
(Figures 3.14 to 3.21)

- Hypercellular smears
- Large cohesive epithelial fragments, with or without three-dimensional papillary architecture and fibrovascular cores; fragments often have scalloped edges
- Often, smaller papillary fragments with intact tips ("anatomic edges")
- Short or tall columnar epithelium, often palisading at the edges of the papilla; nuclear stratification
- Background blood, hemosiderin-laden macrophages
- Significant epithelial atypia (pleomorphism, macronucleoli) may be present

## Pitfalls and Differential Diagnosis

- Papillomas may have significant epithelial proliferation, often with focal cytologic atypia. Careful evaluation with a much higher threshold for carcinoma diagnosis is prudent. This is significantly important in the presence of metaplastic changes or in infarcted papillomas that can harbor significant cytologic atypia (see Figure 3.21).
- Fibroadenoma
- Papillary carcinoma (in situ and invasive)

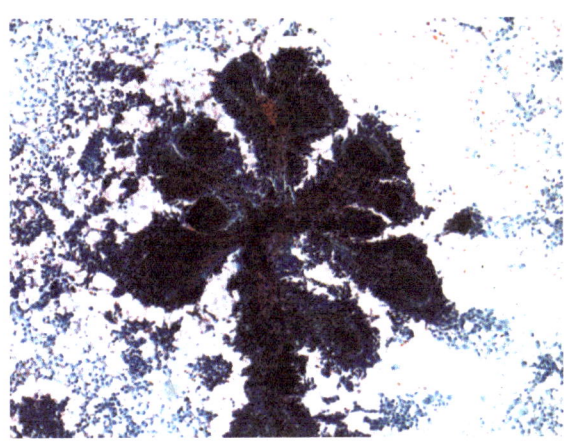

FIGURE 3.14. Intraductal papilloma. Hypercellular smear with a large fragment of ductal epithelium displaying well-formed papillary architecture. The fibrovascular cores covered by layers of proliferative ductal epithelium so characteristic of a papilloma are seldom seen in routine practice. (Smear, Papanicolaou.)

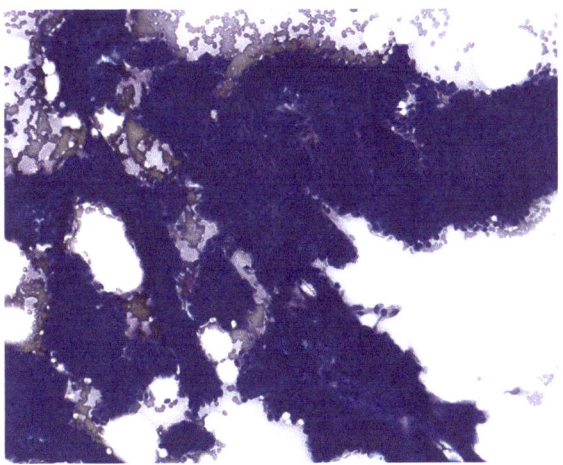

FIGURE 3.15. Intraductal papilloma. Ductal epithelium in an irregularly branched papillary architecture shown here. The epithelial cells appear enlarged, crowded, and disorganized. A well-formed fibrovascular core is often not visualized in these cellular fragments. (Smear, Diff-Quik.)

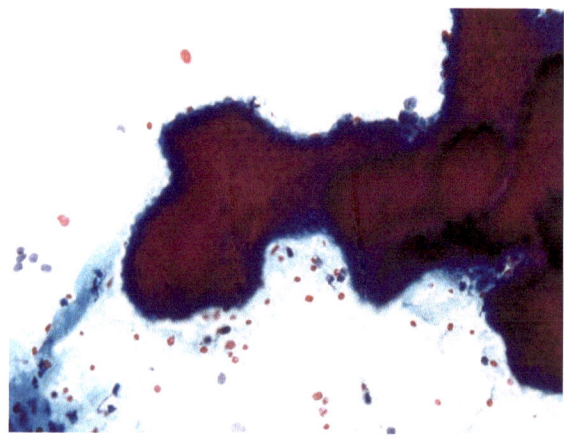

FIGURE 3.16. Intraductal papilloma. Ductal epithelium with a branching papillary architecture is seen. Epithelial cells at the periphery show a palisading of the nuclei. A few myoepithelial cell nuclei are present in the background. (Smear, Papanicolaou.)

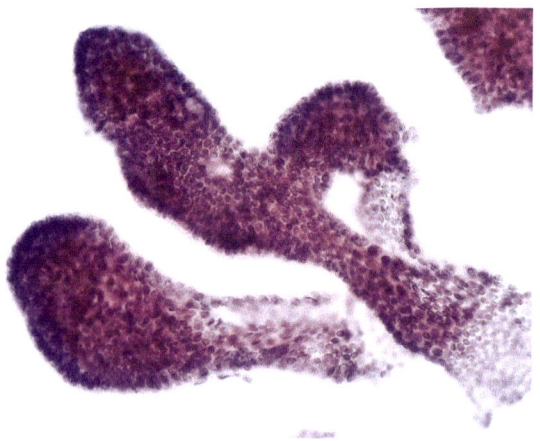

FIGURE 3.17. Intraductal papilloma. Ductal epithelium in a well-formed papillary architecture displays a peculiar palisading of nuclei at the edges. Note the absence of any fibrovascular cores and myo-epithelial cell nuclei in the background. (Smear, Diff-Quik.)

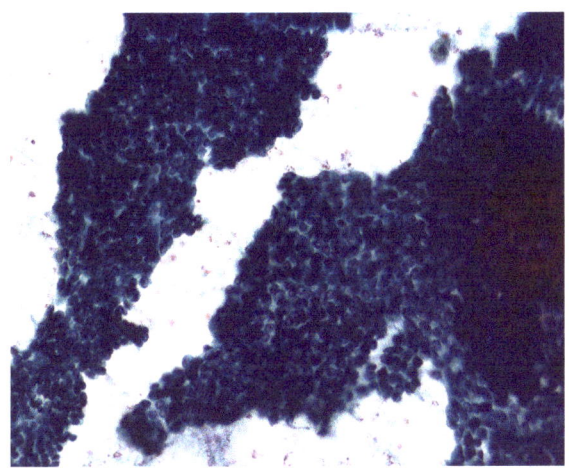

FIGURE 3.18. Intraductal papilloma. Two enlarged fragments of hyperchromatic crowded epithelium appear cytologically atypical. However, a closer look shows the presence of myoepithelial cells and a total lack of singly dispersed atypical epithelial cells. Papillomas may harbor significant epithelial atypia, and one needs to have a significantly higher threshold for interpretation of malignancy in such settings. (Smear, Papanicolaou.)

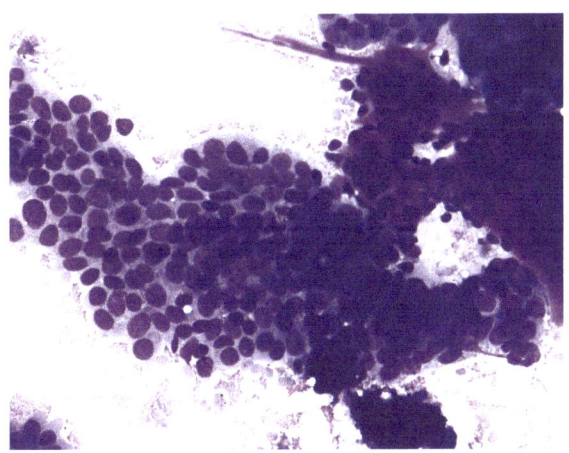

FIGURE 3.19. Intraductal papilloma. Higher magnification shows the degree of epithelial atypia in such lesions. The nuclei are enlarged and pleomorphic. However, there were no individually dispersed epithelial cells in the smear background. (Smear, Diff-Quik.)

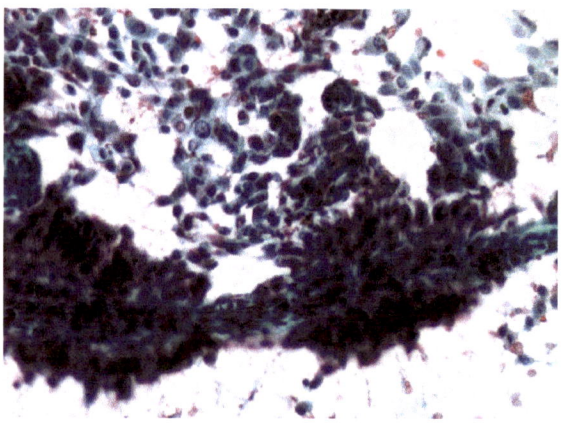

FIGURE 3.20. Intraductal papilloma. Cytologically atypical epithelium uniformly arranged around a fibrovascular core. Numerous, loosely cohesive atypical epithelial cells are seen in the background, admixed with myoepithelial cells. This case was called atypical and turned out to be a papilloma on follow-up resection. (Smear, Papanicolaou.)

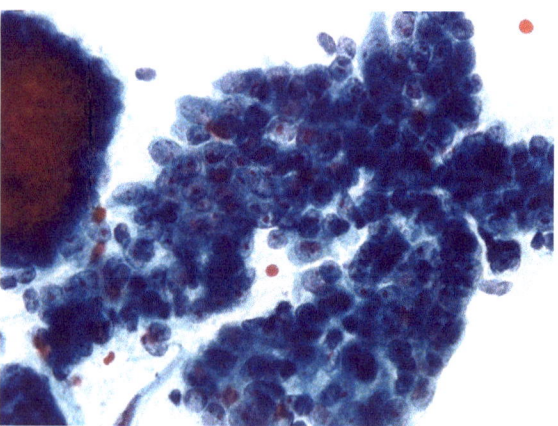

FIGURE 3.21. Intraductal papilloma. Higher magnification shows the extreme degree of cytologic atypia that can be seen in such lesions. The epithelial cells display enlarged, crowded, and pleomorphic nuclei that are totally disorganized and show prominent nucleoli. Rare myoepithelial cell nuclei are also present. (Smear, Papanicolaou.)

# Breast Lesions Diagnosed as "Papillary" on Fine-Needle Aspiration

True papillary lesions of the breast comprise a diverse group of benign and malignant entities. A number of studies have shown that most of these turn out to be "non-papillary" on histologic resection (particularly the malignant cases). This, therefore, raises the question, Do we tend to overinterpret "papillary architecture" on FNA? Papillary lesions were considered an "indeterminate" category at the National Cancer Institute–sponsored consensus conference in 1996.

- Benign follow-up (in two thirds of cases)
  - Intraductal papilloma
  - Papillomatosis
  - Fibroadenoma
  - Fibrocystic changes (with papillary hyperplasia)
- Malignant follow-up (one third of cases)
  - Ductal carcinoma (both in situ and invasive)
  - Phyllodes tumor

# Ductal/Nipple Adenoma

Also known as *papillary adenoma*, ductal/nipple adenoma is a benign mass lesion of the nipple with a prominent papillary architecture. Most adenomas present with nipple discharge.

## *Clinical Features*

- This uncommon neoplasm presents as a discrete, sharply circumscribed nodule with a sclerotic stroma. Most ductal adenomas are up to 2 cm in size and are either solitary or multiple but rarely bilateral.

- Ductal/nipple adenomas occur in the fifth to sixth decades of life and most commonly involve small to mid-sized ducts and less commonly arise in the subareolar region.
- Ductal/nipple adenomas are rarely seen in men.

## Cytomorphologic Features

- Limited cytopathologic experience because of the uncommon occurrence of this lesion
- Variable cellularity, more often low
- Cohesive ductal-type epithelial fragments, tubular or fingerlike papillary morphology
- Presence of myoepithelial cells (only in association with epithelial fragments and not in smear background)

## Pitfalls and Differential Diagnosis

- Hypercellularity may lead to an overcall of atypical or, rarely, malignant diagnosis. Presence of somewhat cohesive fragments and well-identified myoepithelial cells is helpful.

# Granular Cell Tumor

Approximately 6%–8% of all granular cell tumors are encountered in the breast. Clinically and radiologically, granular cell tumor closely mimics primary breast carcinoma (hard spiculated mass often fixed to the overlying skin). Therefore, an accurate FNA diagnosis is extremely critical for disease management.

## Clinical Features

- Average age at presentation is 30 years.
- Most tumors measure less than 2 cm.
- Tumors behave in a benign fashion with local excision curative in most cases.

- A malignant counterpart is exceedingly rare, often requiring adjuvant therapy.

## Cytomorphologic Characteristics

- Variable cellularity, often moderate
- Larger cells, polygonal, densely granular cytoplasm
- Round to oval, uniform, slightly eccentric nuclei
- Numerous naked "stripped off" nuclei in a granular smear background
- Single cells or smaller fragments more common than larger tissue fragments
- Immunostaining with S-100 protein can be extremely helpful

## Pitfalls and Differential Diagnosis

- The dissociated nature of the cells with ample amounts of granular cytoplasm may mimic histiocytes or apocrine metaplastic cells (Distinction from fibrocystic changes, however, is not difficult.)
- Metaplastic carcinoma
- Inflammatory myofibroblastic tumor

# Chondroid Syringoma

## Clinical Features

- Chondroid syringoma is also known as *pleomorphic adenoma* or *benign mixed tumor* (morphologically and immunohistochemically resembling salivary gland pleomorphic adenoma). It presents as a well-defined nodular mass with nonulcerated overlying skin, seen predominantly in face, head, and neck.
- This is a rare neoplasm of the breast that morphologically resemblances the analogous tumor occurring in the salivary gland.

- Chondroid syringoma often forms a discrete, firm nodule in the breast and, therefore, clinically and radiologically resembles a fibroadenoma.
- Most tumors are small and may be up to 2 cm in size. They are easily managed by local resection.
- This tumor is often confused with breast cancer clinically, radiologically, and pathologically.

## *Cytomorphologic Characteristics*
(Figures 3.22 and 3.23)

- Hypercellular smears
- Biphasic appearance with cohesive epithelial fragments, stromal mesenchymal tissue, and myoepithelial cells
- Prominent chondromyxoid stroma
- Often stellatelike arrangement of the epithelial cells

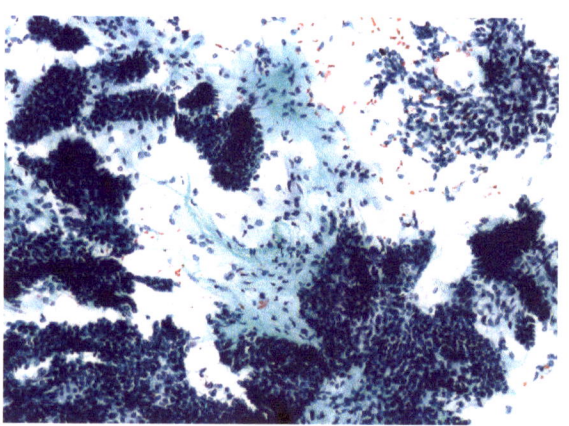

Figure 3.22. Chondroid syringoma. A biphasic population of epithelial fragments and stromal tissue is seen. Cytomorphologic distinction from a fibroadenoma could be difficult if the physical findings in the patient are not known. (Smear, Papanicolaou.)

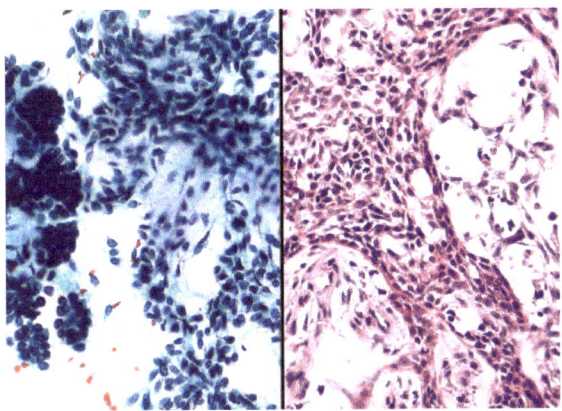

FIGURE 3.23. Chondroid syringoma. A polymorphous appearance of the tumor with nests of epithelium and branching fascicles of spindled cells embedded in a myxoid matrix. Histology of the corresponding tumor is shown on the right. (Smear, Papanicolaou; histologic section, hematoxylin and eosin.)

## *Pitfalls and Differential Diagnosis*

- Fibroadenoma
- Cystosarcoma phyllodes
- Metaplastic carcinoma

# Lipoma

## *Clinical Features*

- Lipomas in the breast are usually subcutaneous and occur most commonly in patients between the ages of 40 and 60 years.
- The patients usually present with a slow-growing soft, solitary mass.
- Lipomas are well circumscribed, sometimes encapsulated, round masses usually less than 5 cm in diameter.

- Some of the variants of lipoma that have been described in the breast include fibrolipoma, angiolipoma, hibernoma, and spindle cell limpoma.

## Cytomorphologic Characteristics

- Hypercellular smears
- Mature adipose tissue

## Differential Diagnosis and Pitfalls

- Fibrocystic changes, papillomatosis

# Myofibroblastoma

## Clinical Features

- Myofibroblastoma is a benign spindle cell neoplasm of breast stroma and is composed of myofibroblasts.
- The patients range in age from 40 to 87 years, with a mean age of 65 years.
- Patients usually present with a slow-growing solitary mass.
- This lesion affects men and women.
- Mammography reveals a relatively well-circumscribed solid mass, usually lacking microcalcifications.

## Cytomorphologic Characteristics

- Predominantly spindle-shaped cells with occasional oval cells
- Spindled myofibroblasts with well-formed nuclear grooves and/or intranuclear inclusions
- Rare mitotic figures
- Desmin-, actin-, and vimentin-positive cells

## Pitfalls and Differential Diagnosis

- Fibrocystic changes, papillomatosis
- Pseudoangiomatous stromal hyperplasia
- Inflammatory myofibroblastic tumor

# Adenomyoepithelioma

## Clinical Features

Adenomyoepithelioma is a rare breast tumor characterized by a biphasic proliferation of epithelial and myoepithelial cells. The tumor has a low malignant potential. Therefore, an accurate FNA diagnosis is clinically important for patient management. The tumor is well-known for its histologic heterogeneity, which is reflected in an often diagnostically difficult cytopathologic interpretation. Three subtypes have been described according to their growth pattern and predominant cell type: tubular, lobular, and spindle. Most cases behave in a benign fashion but can recur locally if incompletely excised. Close follow-up is always required even after excision.

## Cytomorphologic Characteristics
(Figure 3.24 to 3.28)

- Smears are moderate to hypercellular.
- Cohesive fragments of epithelial and myoepithelial cells occur in varying proportions.
- Epithelial cells display cohesive sheets and rarely tubules with uniform nuclei containing grooves.
- Myoepithelial cells have a variegated appearance with spindle, epithelioid, clear cell, and plasmacytoid morphology. They appear as cohesive fragments, single cells with well-preserved clear and vacuolated "soap bubble" cytoplasm, or as naked bipolar nuclei in the background. Occasional intranuclear inclusions are seen.

- Rarely epithelial fragments have an outer layer of cells with clear vacuolated cytoplasm. However, epithelial-myoepithelial distinction is rarely appreciated within the same fragment.
- Background naked bipolar nuclei and metachromatic fibro-myxoid stroma are present (some resemblance to salivary gland–type tumors).
- Stroma may have "collagenous spherulosislike" appearance.
- Rarely, apocrine cells and foamy macrophages are present.
- The tubular variant may show pseudopapillary cores with cells arranged around branching vessels.

## *Pitfalls and Differential Diagnosis*

- Biphasic breast tumors (fibroadenoma and others)
- Low-grade ductal carcinoma
- Mesenchymal neoplasms (of the spindle cell variant)

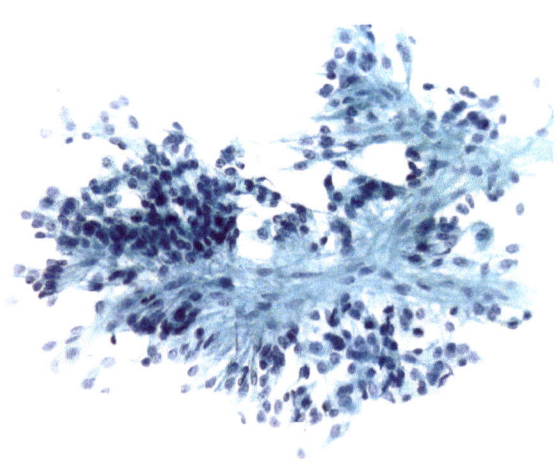

FIGURE 3.24. Adenomyoepithelioma. Loosely cohesive fragment of ductal epithelium surrounding fibrous and myxomatous cores characterize this lesion. (Smear, Papanicolaou.)

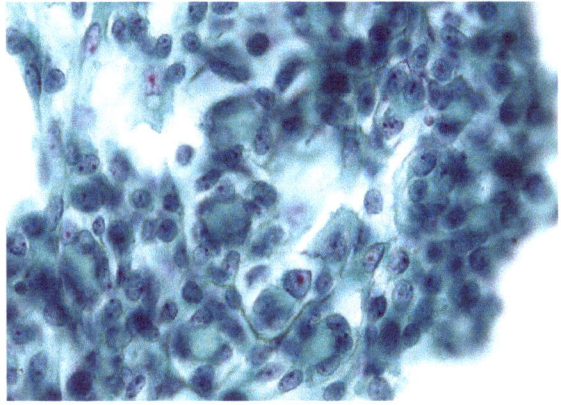

FIGURE 3.25. Adenomyoepithelioma. Fragment of focally atypical epithelium with somewhat enlarged crowded nuclei and focal tubular/glandular architecture (6 o'clock). The cytoplasm is pale to clear with well-defined borders. (Smear, Papanicolaou.).

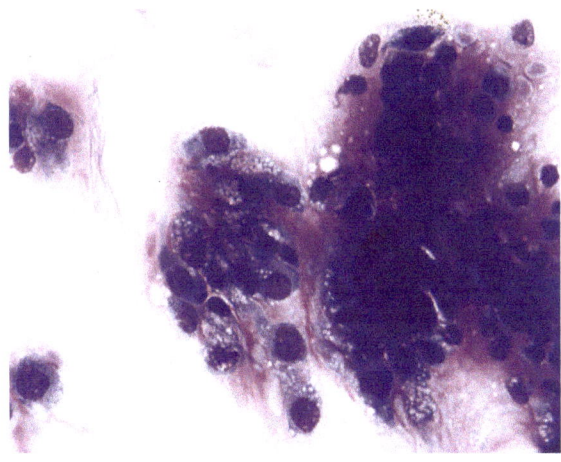

FIGURE 3.26. Adenomyoepithelioma. Higher magnification of somewhat pleomorphic epithelial/myoepithelial cells with the characteristic "soap bubble" cytoplasmic artifact is depicted. The cells are seen in close association with bright magenta-colored stromal material. (Smear, Papanicolaou.)

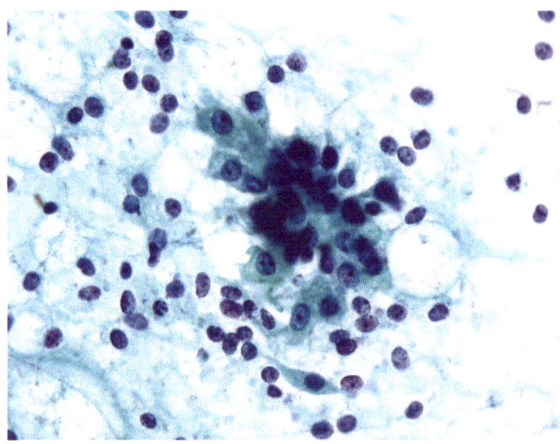

FIGURE 3.27. Adenomyoepithelioma. Higher magnification of a case displaying abundance of naked myoepithelial cell nuclei. (Smear, Papanicolaou.)

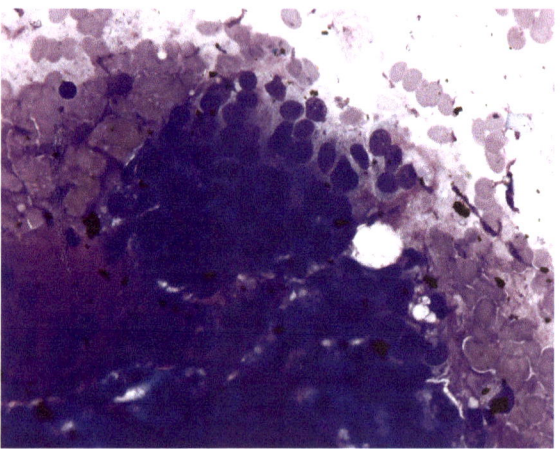

FIGURE 3.28. Adenomyoepithelioma. Higher magnification of a case displaying significant epithelial atypia is shown. There is cellular disorganization with enlarged, crowded, and hyperchromatic nuclei. Cytologic interpretation of this tumor can be extremely difficult, and the cytologic atypia may lead to a false-positive interpretation. (Smear, Diff-Quik.)

# Hamartoma

Hamartoma is a rare tumorlike growth of mature breast tissue lacking structural organization, originally described by Pryn in 1928. Breast hamartoma is considered a dysgenetic rather than a neoplastic disorder. Association with other dysgenetic disorders (such as Cowden syndrome) has been described.

## Clinical Features

- Lesions are well-circumscribed, benign, and composed of fat, glandular tissue, and fibrous connective tissue.
- The majority occur in women who are premenopausal.
- Two variants of hamartoma of the breast have been described: (1) adenolipoma, which is composed of mature adipose tissue with varying amounts of normal breast tissue; and (2) chondrolipoma, which has mature adipose tissue admixed with hyaline cartilage.

## Cytomorphologic Characteristics

- Moderate cellularity
- Irregularly branching sheets of cohesive ductal epithelium
- Intact lobular units
- Lack of cytologic atypia and lack of cellular dispersal
- Abundant naked bipolar nuclei, few stromal fragments, multinucleated histiocytes, rare apocrine cells
- Adipose tissue fragments

## Pitfalls and Differential Diagnosis

- Normal breast tissue
- Fibroadenoma
- Fibrocystic changes

## Selected Reading

Dawson AE, Mulford DK: Benign versus malignant papillary neoplasms of the breast. diagnostic clues in fine needle aspiration cytology. Acta Cytol 1994, 38:23–28.

Gupta RK, McHutchison AG, Dowle CS, Simpson JS: Fine-needle aspiration cytodiagnosis of breast masses in pregnant and lactating women and its impact on management. Diagn Cytopathol 1993, 9:156–159.

Jain S, Kumar N, Sodhani P, Gupta S: Cytology of collagenous spherulosis of the breast: a diagnostic dilemma–report of three cases. Cytopathology 2002, 13:116–120.

Jayaram G, Sthaneshwar P: Fine-needle aspiration cytology of phyllodes tumors. Diagn Cytopathol 2002, 26:222–227.

Lopez-Ferrer P, Jimenez-Heffernan JA, Vicandi B, Ortega L, Viguer JM: Fine needle aspiration cytology of breast fibroadenoma. A cytohistologic correlation study of 405 cases. Acta Cytol 1999, 43:579–586.

Ng WK: Adenomyoepithelioma of the breast. A review of three cases with reappraisal of the fine needle aspiration biopsy findings. Acta Cytol 2002, 46:317–324.

Simsir A, Tsang P, Greenebaum E: Additional mimics of mucinous mammary carcinoma: fibroepithelial lesions. Am J Clin Pathol 1998, 109:169–172.

Simsir A, Waisman J, Cangiarella J: Fibroadenomas with atypia: causes of under- and overdiagnosis by aspiration biopsy. Diagn Cytopathol 2001, 25:278–284.

Stanley MW, Tani EM, Skoog L: Fine-needle aspiration of fibroadenomas of the breast with atypia: a spectrum including cases that cytologically mimic carcinoma. Diagn Cytopathol 1990, 6:375–382.

# 4
# Primary Malignant Tumors

This chapter focuses on primary malignant tumors of the breast, including ductal, lobular, and special types of carcinomas and sarcomas.

## Ductal Carcinoma

This section focuses on the cytomorphology of in situ versus invasive ductal carcinoma. It is emphasized that this represents a difficult area in cytology, and there is significant controversy as to whether it is possible to distinguish between these two types of lesions using only cytomorphology.

### *Ductal Carcinoma In Situ*

Clinical Features

- Accounts for 10%–20% of mammographically detected breast carcinomas
- Arises from terminal duct lobular units

Cytomorphologic Characteristics (Figures 4.1 to 4.9)

- Smears are hypercellular, with sheets and cords of malignant cells.
- Cells are crowded and enlarged. Nuclei are hyperchromatic with occasional prominent nucleoli.

- Myoepithelial cells are lacking.
- The *cribriform* type is characterized by cohesive sheetlike fragments of bland cells with sharply punched out holes. The *micropapillary* form is characterized by abundant large cellular fragments with slender, well-formed papillary structures with narrow avascular stalks and wide bulbous ends. The *comedo* type is characterized by degenerated/ necrotic cellular debris, microcalcifications, foamy macrophages, and pleomorphic malignant cells with a high nuclear grade. The *cystic hypersecretory* type is characterized by pleomorphic cells with cytoplasmic vacuoles and often hobnailed nuclei associated with foamy macrophages, hemosiderin-laden macrophages, cellular debris, and fragments of amorphous colloid-like material.
- A cytopathologic distinction between ductal carcinoma in situ and invasive ductal carcinoma is not possible in most of the cases. Therefore, traditionally both forms of cancers are grouped under the broad cytologic category of "mammary carcinoma."

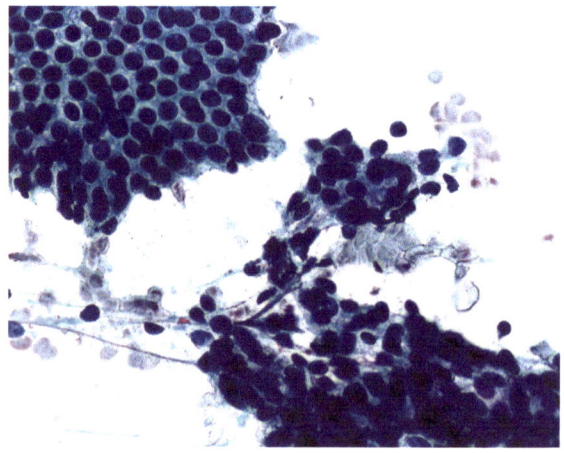

FIGURE 4.1. Ductal carcinoma. Pleomorphic, hyperchromatic malignant cells are seen in a disorganized architecture. A few single malignant cells are present as well. Follow-up biopsy revealed ductal carcinoma in situ, comedo type. (Smear, Papanicolaou.)

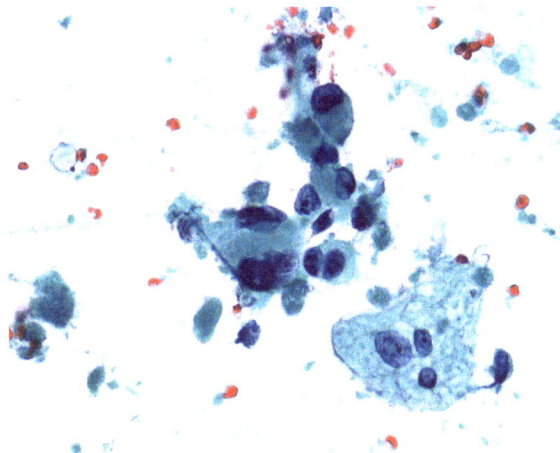

FIGURE 4.2. Ductal carcinoma. Higher magnification shows markedly pleomorphic malignant cells in a loose cluster. Background shows granular necrosis and a few macrophages. Follow-up biopsy revealed ductal carcinoma in situ, comedo type (Smear, Papanicolaou.)

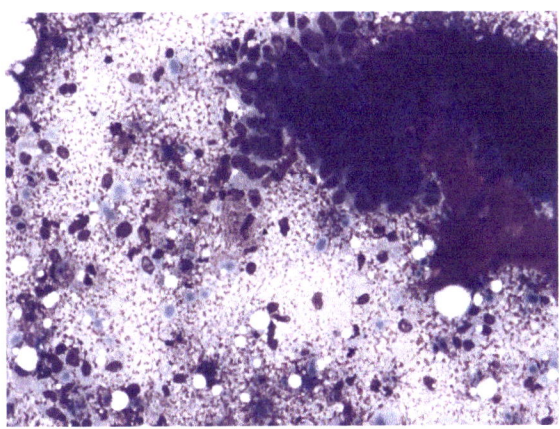

FIGURE 4.3. Ductal carcinoma. A fragment of pleomorphic malignant cells in a background of prominent necrosis. Numerous single malignant cells are seen as well. Follow-up biopsy revealed ductal carcinoma in situ, comedo type. However, a distinction from infiltrating ductal carcinoma could not have been possible with fine-needle aspiration. (Smear, Diff-Quik.)

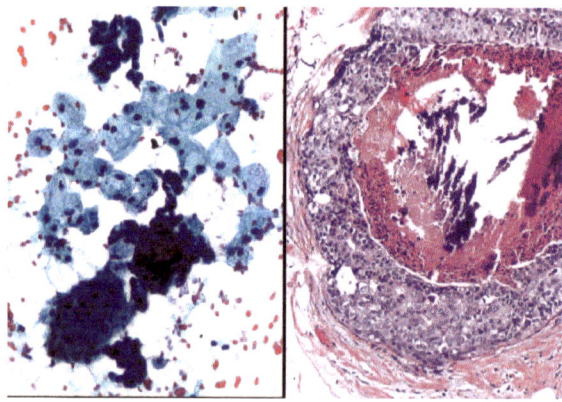

FIGURE 4.4. Ductal carcinoma. Cohesive fragments of ductal carcinoma seen in the background of numerous macrophages and focal
necrosis **(left)**. Follow-up biopsy revealed ductal carcinoma in situ,
comedo type **(right)**. (Smear, Papanicolaou; histologic section,
hematoxylin and eosin.)

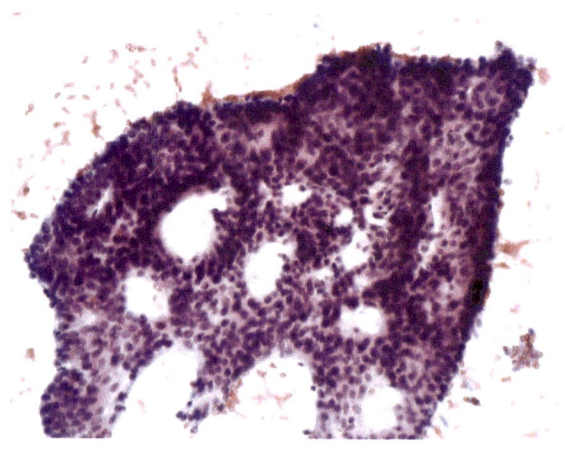

FIGURE 4.5. Ductal carcinoma. A large tissue fragment of malignant
cells with sharply punched out spaces. Follow-up biopsy revealed
ductal carcinoma in situ, cribriform type. (Smear, Diff-Quik.)

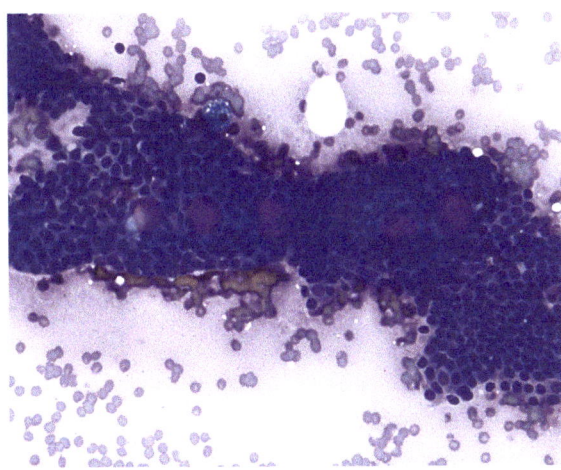

FIGURE 4.6. Ductal carcinoma. Malignant cells seen in a large cohesive fragment with well-formed luminal spaces containing metachromatic material. One of the diagnostic considerations would be an adenoid cystic carcinoma. Follow-up biopsy revealed ductal carcinoma in situ, cribriform type. (Smear, Diff-Quik.)

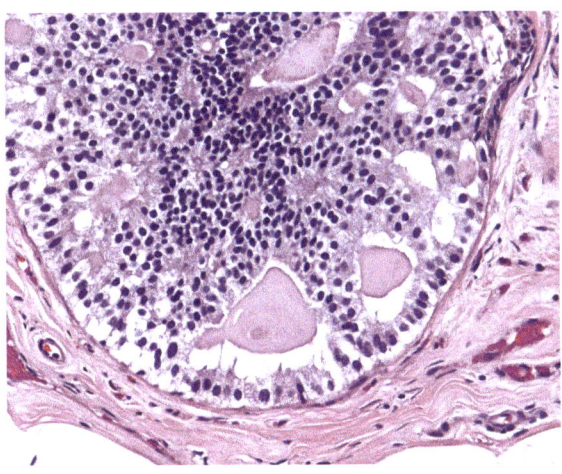

FIGURE 4.7. Ductal carcinoma in situ, cribriform type. Histologic section illustrating eosinophilic amorphous secretions within the cribriform spaces, the likely source of the metachromatic structures seen in Figure 4.6. (Histologic section, hematoxylin and eosin.)

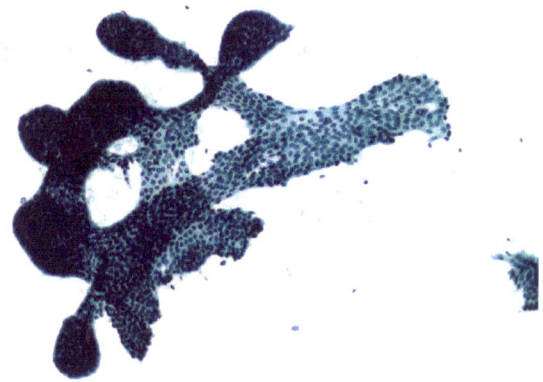

FIGURE 4.8. Ductal carcinoma. A large tissue fragment composed of ductal epithelium with well-formed papillary architecture. The papillae grow as slender projections with round bulbous endings. Because of the low-grade morphology, a distinction from a benign papillary lesion would be extremely difficult. Follow-up tissue biopsy revealed ductal carcinoma in situ, micropapillary type. (Smear, Papanicolaou.)

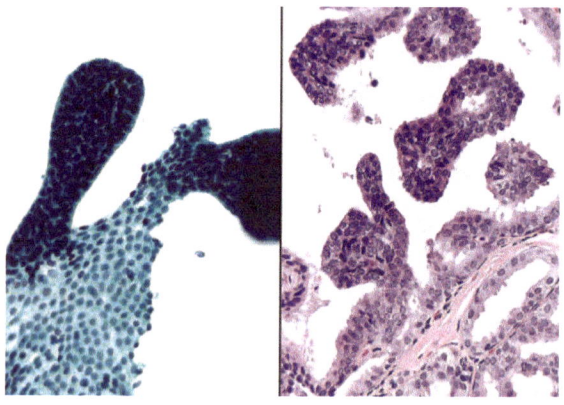

FIGURE 4.9. Ductal carcinoma. Higher magnification shows a well-formed papillary structure projecting from a broad base. Malignant cells have uniform but hyperchromatic nuclei **(left)**. A histologic section of the resected ductal carcinoma in situ, micropapillary type, shows concordant histologic features **(right)**. (Smear, Papanicolaou; histologic section, hematoxylin and eosin.)

Pitfalls and Differential Diagnosis

- Atypical ductal hyperplasia
- Fibroadenoma
- Papilloma/ papillomatosis

## Invasive Ductal Carcinoma Not Otherwise Specified

### Clinical Features

Infiltrating duct cell carcinoma not otherwise specified (NOS) is the most common primary carcinoma of the breast, ranging from 70% to 80% of all breast carcinomas. It is a heterogeneous group of tumors that lack characteristics that would allow their classification as a specific histologic subtype, such as lobular carcinoma. It occurs most frequently in middle-aged to elderly women and rarely in males. These tumors are rare in women younger than 40 years of age. Infiltrating duct cell carcinoma may present as a palpable or nonpalpable breast mass that may or may not demonstrate clinical signs of skin and/or nipple involvement. Possible clinical presentations include hard, fixed mass, "peau d' orange" skin change, ulceration, bloody nipple discharge, and inverted or retracted nipple. Breast carcinoma may also be a solely image-detected lesion. These lesions can be stellate in appearance or well circumscribed.

Mammographically, the vast majority of these malignancies present with a poorly defined spiculated mass with or without microcalcifications. Sonographically, the most common features of malignancy are those of a hypoechoic mass with irregular borders and an uneven echo texture.

Some of the risk factors for breast carcinoma include an early menarche, late menopause, diet high in saturated fat, family history of breast cancer, nulliparity, late first live birth, and first-degree relative with breast cancer. Mutations of the BRCA1 and BRCA2 genes are associated with familial breast cancer at an early age.

Histologic Features

Histologically, infiltrating duct cell carcinoma is characterized by a spectrum of changes that vary according to the atypia and differentiation, such as the degree of tubule formation, nuclear pleomorphism, and mitotic activity. Cytologically, variable patterns reflecting the diverse histologic morphology of the tumors are seen. Breast aspirates of infiltrating duct cell carcinoma are cellular and often show conspicuous loss of cell cohesion.

Cytomorphologic Characteristics (Figures 4.10 to 4.17)

- Variably cellular
- Fragments and singly dispersed malignant cells
- Often a prominent plasmacytoid cellular appearance
- Occasionally, pleomorphism, hyperchromasia, mitosis, necrosis, and a background of tumor diathesis

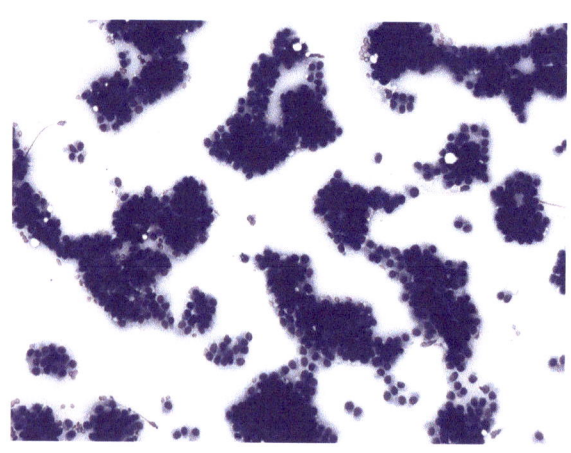

FIGURE 4.10. Ductal carcinoma. Irregular fragments of carcinoma with enlarged, hyperchromatic nuclei. A few single malignant cells are noted as well. A follow-up biopsy revealed an infiltrating ductal carcinoma. (Smear, Diff-Quik.)

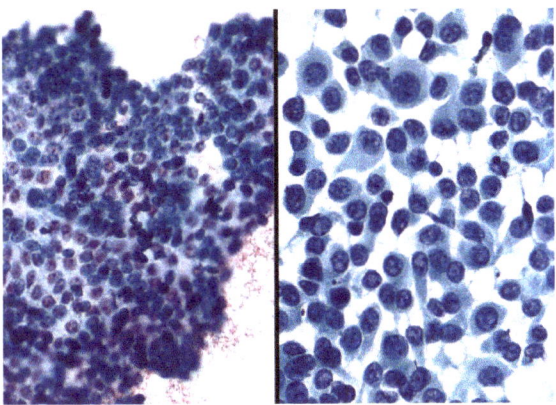

FIGURE 4.11. Ductal carcinoma and atypical ductal hyperplasia. Compare and contrast cytomorphologic characteristics of these two entities. Infiltrating ductal carcinoma **(right)** shows greater pleomorphism, a significantly large nuclear size, more cellular dissociation, and prominent eccentric placement of the nucleus than atypical ductal hyperplasia **(left)**. (Smear, Papanicolaou.)

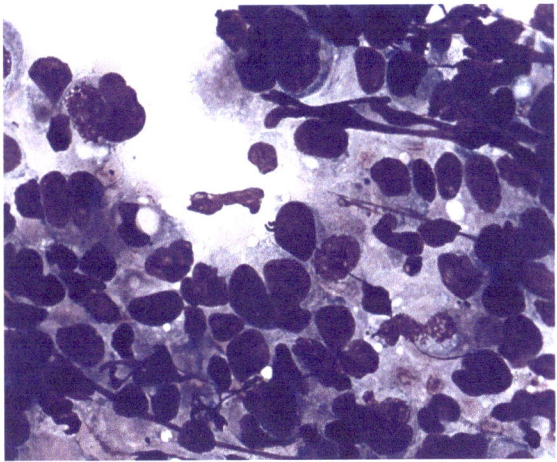

FIGURE 4-12. Ductal carcinoma. Higher magnification of the tumor with overt malignant characteristics, that is, dissociated cells, marked nuclear enlargement, nuclear hyperchromasia, and a totally disorganized architecture. A follow-up biopsy revealed an infiltrating ductal carcinoma. (Smear, Diff-Quik.)

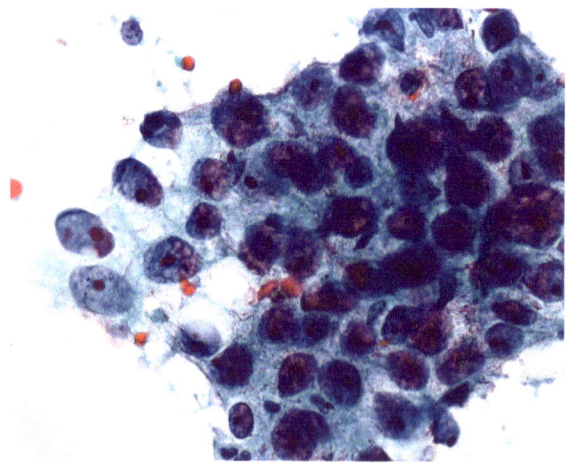

FIGURE 4.13. Ductal carcinoma. Higher magnification of malignant cells with pleomorphic, enlarged nuclei in a syncytial aggregate. Nuclei have macronucleoli, a feature uncommonly seen in classic ductal carcinoma. A follow-up biopsy revealed an infiltrating ductal carcinoma. (Smear, Papanicolaou.)

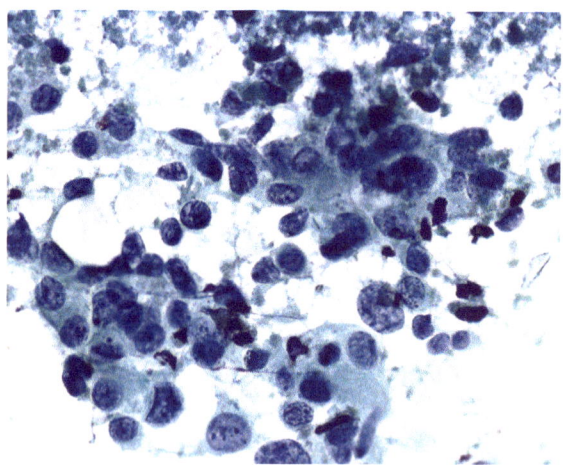

FIGURE 4.14. Ductal carcinoma. Higher magnification of the high-grade tumor with markedly pleomorphic cells. The cells are scattered, often displaying naked nuclei in a necrotic background. A follow-up biopsy revealed an infiltrating ductal carcinoma. (Smear, Papanicolaou.)

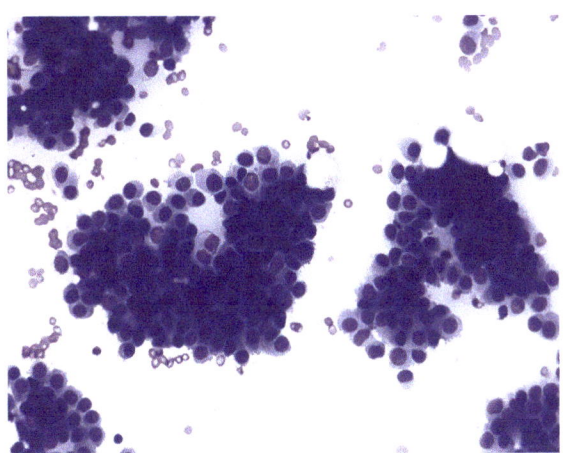

FIGURE 4.15. Ductal carcinoma. A well-differentiated tumor with relatively uniform "plasmacytoid" cells loosely arranged as irregular fragments. A follow-up biopsy revealed an infiltrating ductal carcinoma. (Smear, Diff-Quik.)

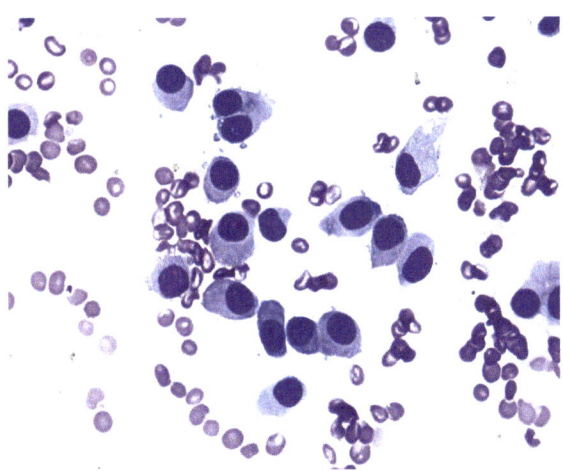

FIGURE 4.16. Ductal carcinoma. Higher magnification shows a loose cluster of malignant cells with round uniform nuclei, eccentrically placed in the cell cytoplasm. A follow-up biopsy revealed an infiltrating ductal carcinoma. (Smear, Diff-Quik.)

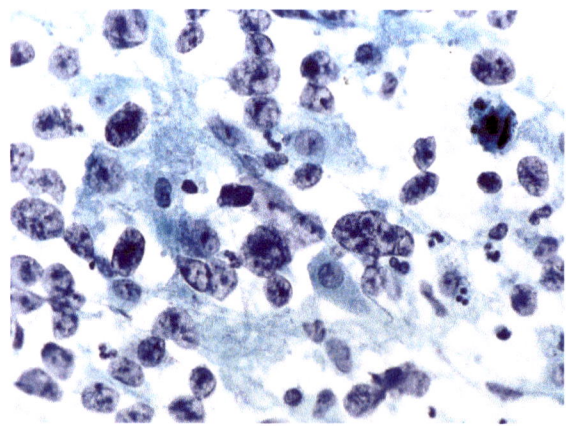

FIGURE 4.17. Ductal carcinoma. A high-grade pleomorphic tumor with singly dispersed naked nuclei. The nuclei are pleomorphic with prominent irregularity of the membrane and devoid of nucleoli. A follow-up biopsy revealed an infiltrating ductal carcinoma. (Smear, Papanicolaou.)

Pitfalls and Differential Diagnosis

- Atypical ductal hyperplasia (see Figure 4.11)
- Fibroadenoma
- Papilloma/papillomatosis
- Lobular carcinoma
- Metastatic cancers

# Lobular Carcinoma

## Lobular Carcinoma In Situ

Clinical Features

- Usually an incidental pathologic finding because it does not form a palpable or mammographically detectable lesion

- Seen in premenopausal age
- Multicentric and often bilateral
- Often associated with atypical lobular hyperplasia
- Increased risk of developing invasive carcinoma

Cytomorphologic Characteristics (Figures 4.18 and 4.19)

- Moderately cellular
- Epithelial fragments, often depicting intact lobular structures
- Myoepithelial cell layer present around the intact neoplastic lobules
- Small cells, tightly packed with monomorphic round nuclei, scant cytoplasm
- Intracytoplasmic vacuoles or lumina, sometimes with targetoid mucin vacuoles
- Because the cytopathologic features of lobular carcinoma in situ are often shared with invasive lobular carcinoma,

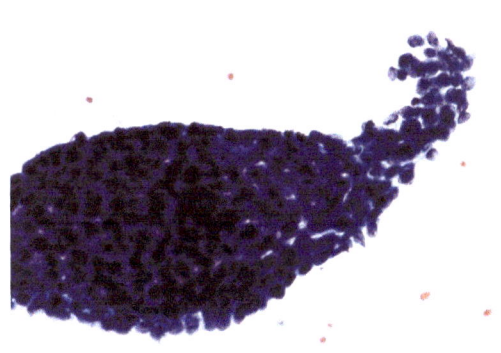

FIGURE 4.18. Lobular carcinoma. A well-formed, cohesive fragment of uniform hyperchromatic malignant cells. A lobular architecture is clearly evident. A follow-up biopsy revealed lobular carcinoma in situ. (Smear, Papanicolaou.)

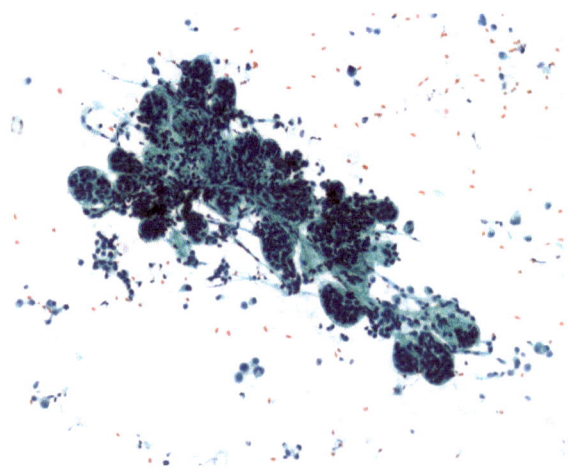

FIGURE 4.19. Lobular carcinoma. Malignant cells seen in an intact lobular architecture as well as singly in the smear background. A follow-up biopsy procedure revealed in situ and infiltrating lobular carcinoma. (Smear, Papanicolaou.)

the distinction between in situ and invasive lobular neoplasia should not be attempted with FNA

Pitfalls and Differential Diagnosis
- Atypical lobular hyperplasia
- Pregnancy/lactational changes

## Invasive Lobular Carcinoma

Clinical Features

Infiltrating lobular carcinoma is diagnosed in approximately 7%–10% of primary breast carcinomas. It occurs in a wide range of age groups, ranging from 26 to 86 years. Clinical presentation is similar to those of other primary breast carcinomas; however, it is not associated with Paget's disease, and occasionally it may present as an indurated area without any discrete mass. Infiltrating lobular carcinoma has a different pattern of metastatic presentation and tends to involve skeletal, visceral, serosal, and meningeal areas. Similarly, ovary, bone, and uterus are the common sites of metastasis from this tumor.

Mammographically, it can present as an asymmetric density with no clearly delineated margin with no or little architectural distortion. A mass may be firm to hard or not readily palpable or visible. The mass may be detected mammographically, although microcalcifications are uncommon. Multifocal infiltrating lobular carcinoma may present with minimal distortion with no significant mass or increased density. These subtle mammographic features warrant careful examination of the breast and sampling of any suspicious area. Infiltrating lobular carcinoma is often bilateral and shows evidence of multicentricity.

Histologic Features

Pathologically, infiltrating lobular carcinoma is characterized by diffuse infiltration of mammary stroma and ductal structures by neoplastic cells in a pagetoid growth pattern. The tumor may be difficult to define by gross examination because of the diffuse nature of the malignancy. Areas of carcinoma in situ are commonly seen. Histologic growth patterns of lobular carcinoma include solid, alveolar, and the pleomorphic variant.

This variety of patterns exhibits similar prognostic behavior except the pleomorphic variant, which is associated with a more unfavorable outcome. By immunohistochemistry, a majority of the lobular carcinomas (up to 95%) are estrogen receptor positive, while 60%–70% are progesterone receptor positive. Immunohistochemical analysis has shown a complete loss of E-cadherin expression in a majority of infiltrating lobular carcinomas (80%–100%).

Cytomorphologic Characteristics (Figures 4.19 to 4.25)

- Lesions have variable cellularity, and smears are usually hypercellular.
- Cells have small uniform nuclei and small nucleoli.

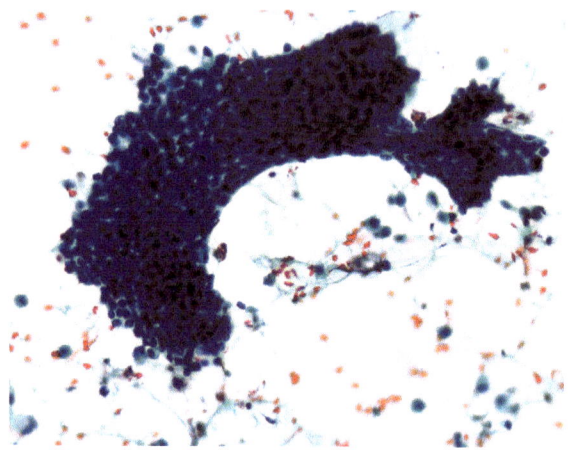

FIGURE 4.20. Lobular carcinoma. A large lobular fragment tightly packed with small, uniform, hyperchromatic nuclei. Numerous single carcinoma cells are evident in the smear background. A follow-up biopsy procedure revealed in situ and infiltrating lobular carcinoma. (Smear, Papanicolaou.)

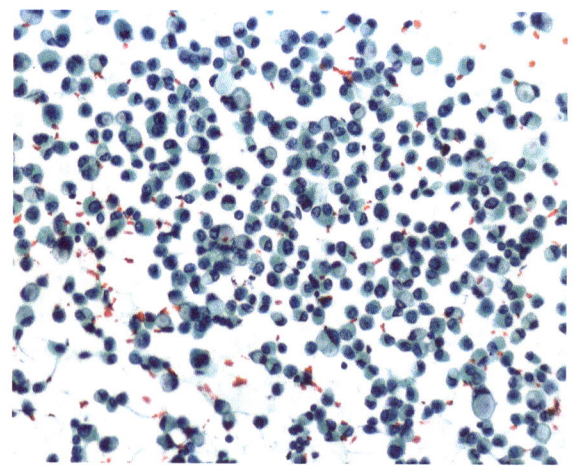

FIGURE 4.21. Lobular carcinoma. A diffusely dispersed population of small and uniform malignant cells with eccentrically placed nuclei and well-defined cytoplasmic vacuoles containing targetoid inclusions. (Smear, Papanicolaou.)

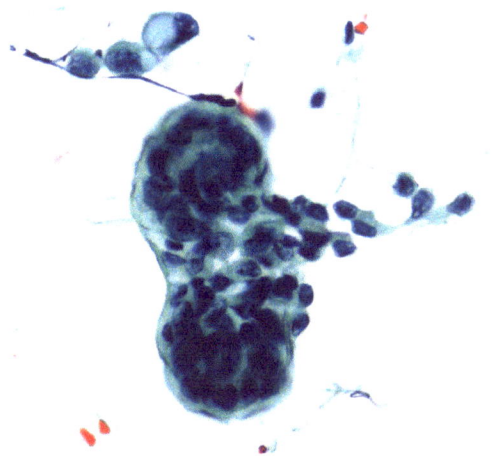

FIGURE 4.22. Lobular carcinoma. Higher magnification of a partially intact neoplastic breast nodule tightly packed with small, round, hyperchromatic nuclei. Few isolated carcinoma cells are seen in the background, one with a well-defined cytoplasmic vacuole. (Smear, Papanicolaou.)

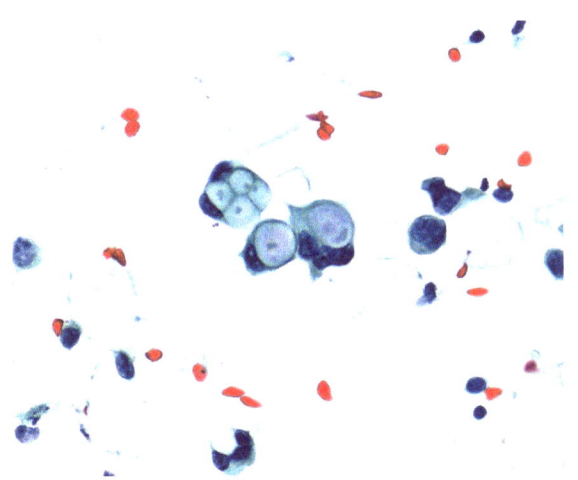

FIGURE 4.23. Lobular carcinoma. Higher magnification shows single and multiple cytoplasmic vacuoles containing targetoid mucin inclusions. Cells have a signet ring morphology with a few mimicking benign lymphocytes. (Smear, Papanicolaou.)

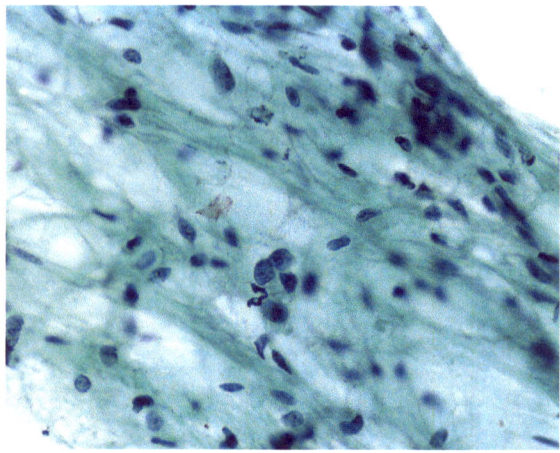

FIGURE 4.24. Lobular carcinoma. A dense fragment of fibrous tissue containing deceptively bland-appearing carcinoma cells. The cytopathologic diagnosis of lobular carcinoma is often difficult because of the absence of classic malignant features and inconspicuous infiltration of malignant cells. (Smear, Papanicolaou.)

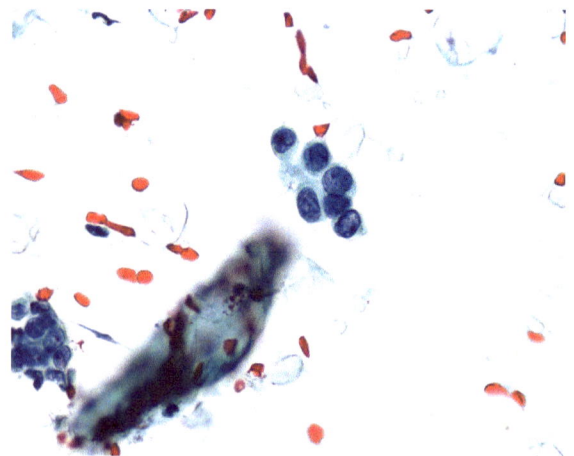

FIGURE 4.25. Lobular carcinoma. A higher magnification shows malignant cells with high nucleus to cytoplasm ratios and barely visible cytoplasm. A casual look at the aspirate may easily mistake such neoplastic cells for benign lymphocytes. (Smear, Papanicolaou.)

- Predominant pattern is that of dissociation; "Indian file" appearance is rarely appreciated in smears.
- Lesions may have little or no atypia.
- Nuclei are eccentric, with occasional intracytoplasmic lumina with mucin droplets and rare signet ring cells.
- Monomorphic pattern of small cells arranged as single cells, cords, or clusters with no recognizable myoepithelial cells are the key features to differentiate infiltrating lobular carcinoma from benign breast lesions.
- The pleomorphic variant features more pleomorphism and nuclear atypia.

### Pitfalls and Differential Diagnosis

Infiltrating lobular carcinoma is one of the main causes of a false-negative diagnosis in breast FNA. This is often due to the minimal atypia associated with this entity.

Differentiation between infiltrating lobular carcinoma versus other entities may be difficult. Especially if the sample is a hypocellular specimen, it is best to consider surgical excision for further characterization of suspicious cells for lobular carcinoma. There are overlapping features among atypical lobular hyperplasia, lobular carcinoma in situ, and an infiltrating lobular carcinoma. These entities are collectively called *lobular neoplasia* if the distinction is not possible.

Higher cellularity and a higher proportion of dissociated cells are commonly seen in an infiltrating lobular carcinoma. Differential diagnosis also includes other low nuclear grade carcinomas of ductal origin. Immunostain for E-cadherin can differentiate between these two entities.

# Special Types of Breast Carcinomas

## *Signet Ring Carcinoma*

### Clinical Features

- These rare breast tumors are associated with an unfavorable prognosis.

- They represent 2%–4% of all breast carcinomas.
- Lesions occur in patients older than the average age of patients with ordinary breast carcinoma.
- The usual age is in the mid to late fifties.
- Signet ring cell carcinomas tend to be more aggressive than mucinous/colloid, ductal, and lobular carcinomas.
- Signet ring cell carcinomas tend to involve metastatic sites such as serosal surfaces of the stomach, female genital tract, and urinary tract.
- They tend to have a high incidence of lymph node involvement and advanced stage of presentation. The prognosis is usually poor.
- The origin of this as a variant of mucinous carcinoma versus an infiltrating lobular carcinoma remains controversial, and many cases cited in the literature have been classified as a variant of infiltrating lobular carcinoma.
- These tumors must be distinguished from duct-derived tumors such as colloid and mucinous carcinomas.

Cytomorphologic Characteristics

- The tumor is characterized by infiltration of breast stroma by signet ring cells with an obvious intracellular mucin accumulation.
- Tumors may present with moderate to rich cellularity.
- The cells are arranged singly and in small, loose clusters.
- The cells are small with crescent-shaped nuclei compressed to the cell periphery by mucin.
- The mucin is mucicarmine and periodic acid–Schiff positive and is packed in a cytoplasmic vacuole.

Pitfalls and Differential Diagnosis

- The differential diagnosis includes metastatic carcinoma, especially from gastrointestinal tumors, infiltrating lobular carcinomas, secretory carcinomas, and lipid-secreting carcinomas.
- Clinical history, the original pathology slides, and ancillary studies such as special stains, electron microscopy, and a

panel of immunostaining for organ-specific antibodies are the tools to distinguish between a primary signet ring carcinoma and a metastatic tumor.

- The distinction between signet ring carcinoma and other tumors requires special attention to subtle morphologic differences.
- Infiltrating lobular carcinomas often show other characteristics of this tumor, including (although rare), the presence of the "Indian file" pattern. Secretory carcinomas present with several prominent intracytoplasmic vacuoles.
- Lipid-rich carcinomas contain small cytoplasmic vacuoles that present in different forms. The vacuoles are often seen in the perinuclear area, and nuclei are indented. Special stain demonstrates the presence of fat droplets in the cytoplasm of tumor cells. These droplets are mucin negative.
- Signet ring carcinomas must also be distinguished from colloid/mucinous breast carcinomas because of the variability in the clinical outcomes of these lesions. In signet ring breast carcinomas, the mucin is present intracytoplasmically, whereas in the colloid carcinomas, the tumor is present as clusters of tumor cells in large mucin pools.

## Invasive Micropapillary Carcinoma

Clinical Features

- Invasive micropapillary carcinoma is a rare variant of infiltrating ductal carcinoma first described by Siriaunkgul and Tavassoli in 1993. It is characterized by the presence of small clusters of tumor cells within artificially dilated stromal spaces, the so-called morular or micropapillary growth pattern. Also characteristic is the reverse cellular polarity or the so-called inside-out appearance.
- This type is more frequently seen admixed with invasive ductal carcinoma rather than in its pure form.
- These tumors account for less than 3% of all invasive breast tumors.

- The age group is the same as that for the usual invasive breast carcinomas NOS.
- Patients present with a solid mass.
- This subtype of tumor is associated with vascular invasion and the presence of lymph node metastasis, that is, lymphotropism, skin and chest wall recurrences, advanced stage at presentation, and expression of unfavorable prognostic markers.
- Axillary lymph node metastasis is usually present in about 75% of the patients.

Cytomorphologic Characteristics

- Tumors have distinctive cytomorphologic features.
- There are three-dimensional tissue fragments ("cell balls"), acini, and papillary structures of hyperchromatic cells with crowded nuclei. No fibrovascular cores are present, and there are few single cells.
- The morulae have tightly cohesive malignant cells with smooth, rounded outer borders or "community borders."
- Enlarged hyperchromatic nuclei, prominent nucleoli, and high nucleus to cytoplasm ratios.
- Few cases show prominent apocrine morphology.
- Focal mucinous background can be seen.
- Rare cases have psammoma bodies.
- Apical cytoplasm is toward the periphery, while the nuclei are toward the center in these clusters. The reverse polarity can be demonstrated in cell block sections using epithelial membrane antigen immunostain.
- Blood is often abundant and contains hemosiderin-laden macrophages.

Pitfalls and Differential Diagnosis

- Papilloma, papillomatosis
- Ductal carcinoma in situ, micropapillary type
- Metastatic papillary ovarian serous carcinoma
- Apocrine carcinoma

- Colloid carcinoma
- Fibroadenoma

# Lipid-Rich Carcinoma

Clinical Features

- Lipid-rich carcinoma is an extremely rare variant (1%) of invasive breast carcinoma, characterized by the presence of abundant cytoplasmic neutral lipids in the majority of neoplastic cells of the tumor.
- The patient age range is wide, from 33 to 81 years.
- Most patients present with palpable masses.
- The reported tumor sizes have ranged from 1.2 to 15 cm.
- In a series of 13 cases, described by Ramos et al. in 1974, 11 patients had extensive lymph node metastasis.

Cytomorphologic Characteristics

- Most cases show invasive carcinoma with neoplastic cells with large, foamy, vacuolated cytoplasm.
- The droplets within the cytoplasm contain neutral lipids.

Pitfalls and Differential Diagnosis

- Secretory carcinoma
- Glycogen-rich carcinoma
- Apocrine carcinoma

# Colloid (Mucinous) Carcinoma

Clinical Features

- More common in the postmenopausal age group
- Distinctly better prognosis
- Rarely metastasizes, but often local recurrences occur
- Less nodal involvement than in infiltrating ductal carcinoma NOS
- Often present as a large slowly growing mass, soft and well circumscribed on palpation

- Characteristically, abundant mucin that can be seen grossly

Cytomorphologic Characteristics (Figures 4.26 to 4.29)

- Abundant mucin
- Gelatinous-appearing aspirates
- Loosely cohesive, minimally pleomorphic epithelial fragments
- Occasional single malignant cells
- Cytoplasmic mucin vacuoles
- Fragments of stroma with capillary vessels

Pitfalls and Differential Diagnosis

- Mucocele
- Adenoid cystic carcinoma
- Fibroadenoma showing myxoid change

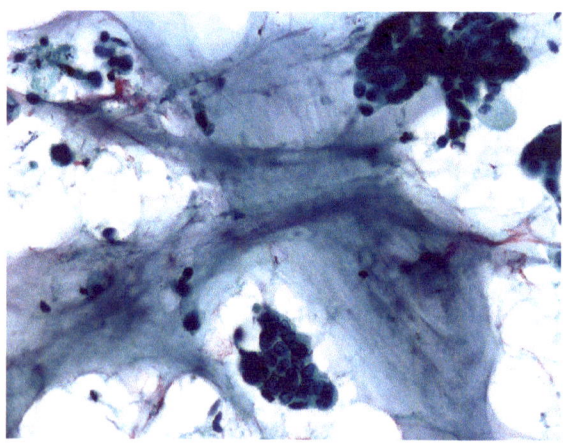

FIGURE 4.26. Colloid carcinoma. Abundant mucin containing a few loosely cohesive fragments of carcinoma cells. The appearance of malignant cells in colloid carcinoma is often low grade, requiring careful exclusion of other benign entities with mucinous features such as mucocele and fibroadenoma with abundant mucinous stroma. (Smear, Papanicolaou.)

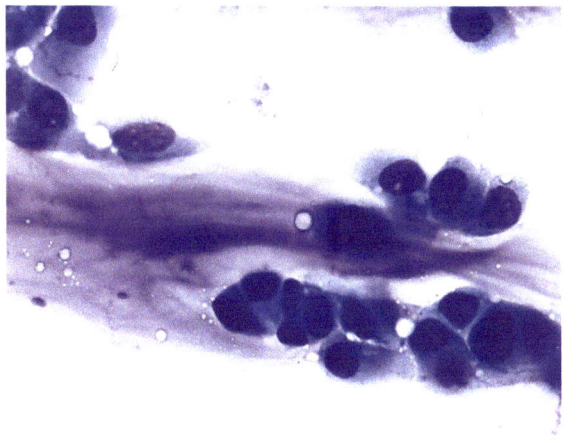

FIGURE 4.27. Colloid carcinoma. Higher magnification shows loosely dispersed malignant cells with large pleomorphic nuclei in a background of abundant mucin. (Smear, Diff-Quik.)

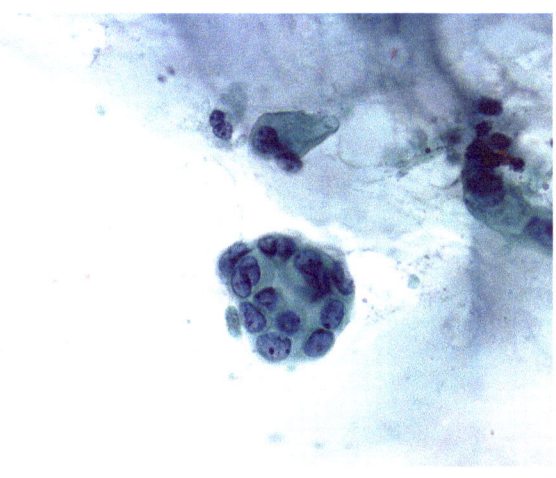

FIGURE 4.28. Colloid carcinoma. A small three-dimensional fragment of ductal carcinoma floating in a mucinous background. (Smear, Papanicolaou.)

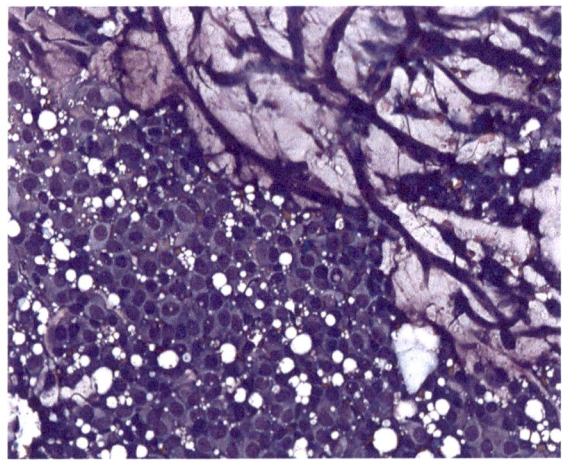

FIGURE 4.29. Colloid carcinoma. An unusual feature of this tumor is the presence of a prominent tangled mass of fine capillaries. Abundant mucin and isolated tumor cells are seen in the background as well. (Smear, Diff-Quik.).

## Tubular Carcinoma

Clinical Features

- This is a well-differentiated subtype of ductal carcinoma, is low grade, and has a distinctly better prognosis.
- The incidence is low, ranging from 1% to 2%.
- The average age at diagnosis is 50 years.
- Cells are commonly multicentric, often bilateral.
- The majority of the tumors are not palpable.
- Mammographically, tumors have an ill-defined, spiculated appearance, similar to a radial scar.
- This type is more commonly seen as a component of invasive ductal carcinoma NOS.

Cytomorphologic Characteristics (Figures 4.30 to 4.33)

- Tumors are composed entirely of complex cords and tubular structures (>75%).
- Cellularity is variable.

- Tumors contain epithelial fragments, usually cohesive, with a prominent tubular architecture.
- Tubules have rigid walls, and the lumen is often open ended with frequent scalloping or right-angle branching.
- Glands have comma-shaped morphology.
- There is minimal atypia and nuclear monomorphism.
- Occasionally, background myoepithelial nuclei are present.
- Fibrous tissue fragments are often densely collagenized.

Pitfalls and Differential Diagnosis

- Fibroadenoma
- Benign ductal epithelium (such as in adenosis)

## Medullary Carcinoma

Clinical Features

- Special type of tumor with syncytial sheets of pleomorphic cells, increased mitoses, lymphocytic infiltrate

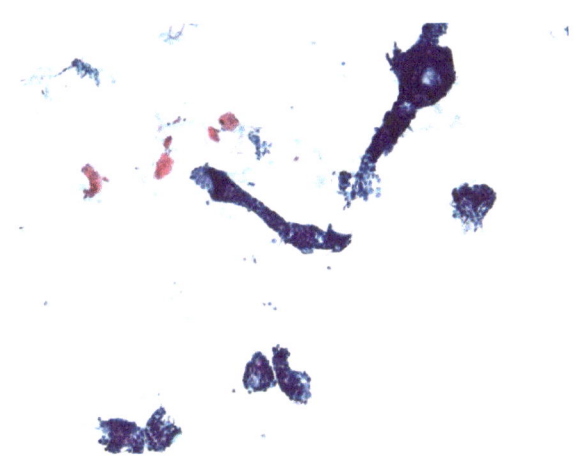

FIGURE 4.30. Tubular carcinoma. Tightly cohesive fragments of carcinoma with a prominent tubular morphology. Note the lack of any background cells, including red blood cells. (Smear, Papanicolaou.)

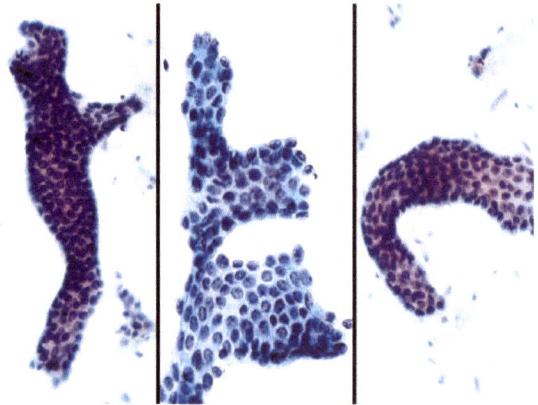

FIGURE 4.31. Tubular carcinoma. This composite image shows a pathognomonic feature of the tumor, that is, formation of a rigid tubular architecture ("hose pipe–like"). Also notice the characteristic right angle branching of the tubules. (Smear, Papanicolaou.)

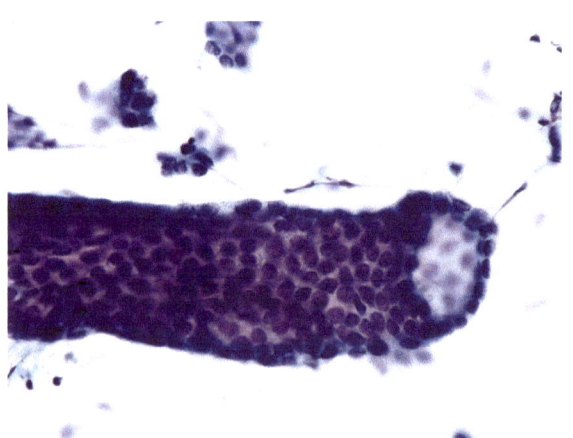

FIGURE 4.32. Tubular carcinoma. Higher magnification of the tubular architecture. The carcinoma cells are uniform and appear low grade. Noticeable features include a rigid architecture with parallel walls and open lumen at the end. (Smear, Papanicolaou.)

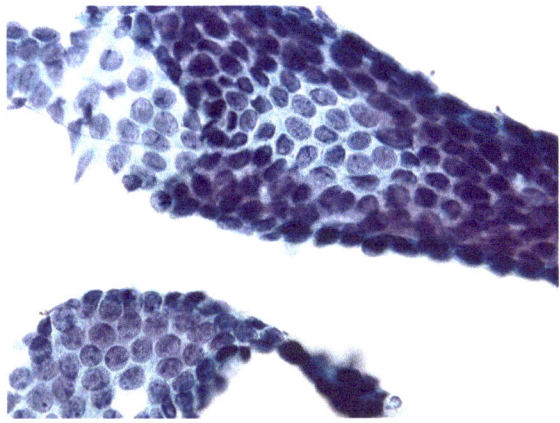

FIGURE 4.33. Tubular carcinoma. The tumor consists of small, round, uniform nuclei arranged in tubules with open lumens and prominent scalloping (noted at 6 o'clock). (Smear, Papanicolaou.)

- More common in younger patients
- Presents as a solitary, soft, well-circumscribed, and mobile mass
- Clinically mimics fibroadenoma, benign cyst, or an intra-mammary lymph node
- Much better prognosis, even with axillary node metastasis

Cytomorphologic Characteristics (Figures 4.34 to 4.37)

- Hypercellular smears
- Relatively larger, pleomorphic cells, single or in loose clusters, often syncytial arrangements
- Large nuclei with large nucleoli
- Naked nuclei with macronucleoli, better appreciated on Diff-Quik stain
- Background lymphocytes, often in close proximity to cellular syncytia
- Cellular degeneration and/or necrosis

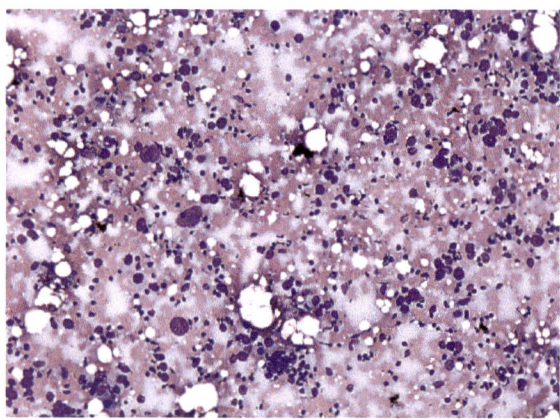

FIGURE 4.34. Medullary carcinoma. Hypercellular smear composed of carcinoma cells and benign lymphocytes. Note the naked nuclear appearance of the malignant cells. (Smear, Diff-Quik.)

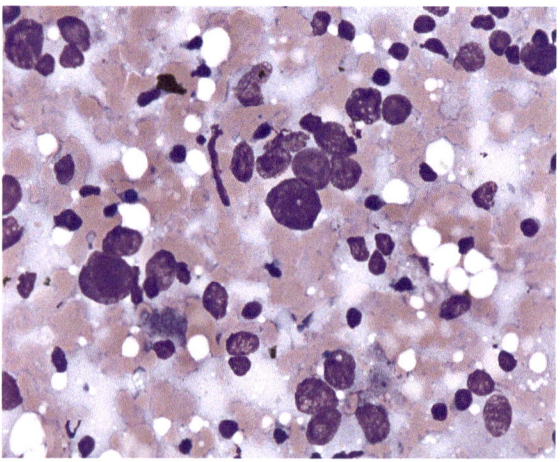

FIGURE 4.35. Medullary carcinoma. Higher magnification shows malignant cells with naked nuclei and macronucleoli intimately admixed with benign lymphocytes. (Smear, Diff-Quik.)

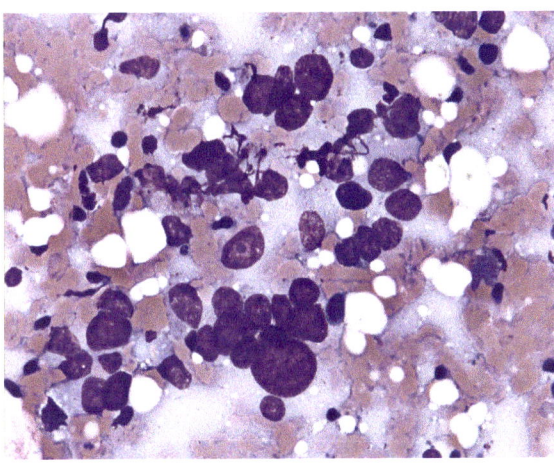

FIGURE 4.36. Medullary carcinoma. Pleomorphic naked nuclei with macronucleoli and rare background lymphocytes. Primary breast carcinomas most often lack macronucleoli with the exception of the rare medullary carcinoma and apocrine carcinoma. (Smear, Diff-Quik.)

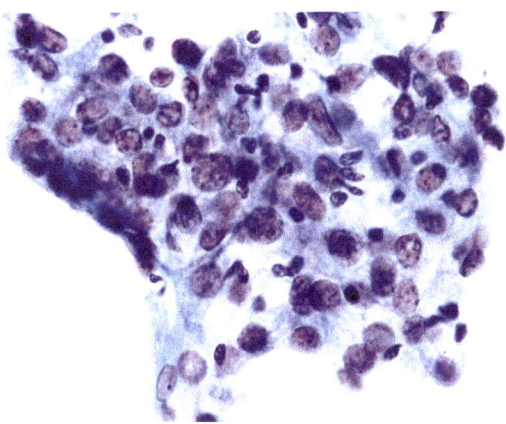

FIGURE 4.37. Medullary carcinoma. A syncytial fragment of pleomorphic malignant cells. Few lymphocytes are visible closely adhering to the fragment. There is a total lack of glandular differentiation in these tumors. (Smear, Papanicolaou.)

Pitfalls and Differential Diagnosis

- Invasive ductal carcinoma NOS

## *Secretory Carcinoma*

Clinical Features

- First reported in children and called *juvenile carcinoma*
- Occurs in children, adolescents, and adults
- Occurs in both men and women
- Shows a tubuloalveolar pattern of growth

Cytomorphologic Characteristics

- Hypercellular smears
- Background mucinous material
- Cells with abundant cytoplasm and intracytoplasmic vacuoles
- "Globules" of secretory material

Pitfalls and Differential Diagnosis

- Fibrocystic changes, papillomatosis
- Lactational changes

## *Adenoid Cystic Carcinoma*

Clinical Features

- Rare tumors with good prognosis
- Slowly enlarging breast mass
- Lobulated and well-defined by mammography

Cytomorphologic Characteristics (Figures 4.38 and 4.39)

- Smears with globules and/or cylinders of pale blue hyaline material on Papanicolaou stain
- Bright magenta globules on Diff-Quik stain
- Small hyperchromatic cells with very little cytoplasm surrounding the globules
- Inconspicuous nucleoli

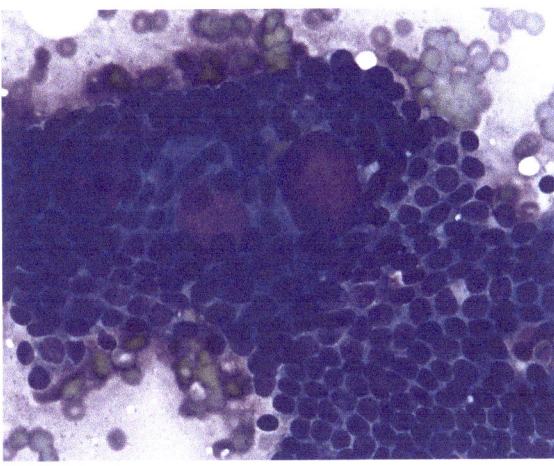

FIGURE 4.38. Adenoid cystic carcinoma. A large fragment of basaloid-type epithelium containing well-defined magenta-colored hyaline globules. (Smear, Diff-Quik.)

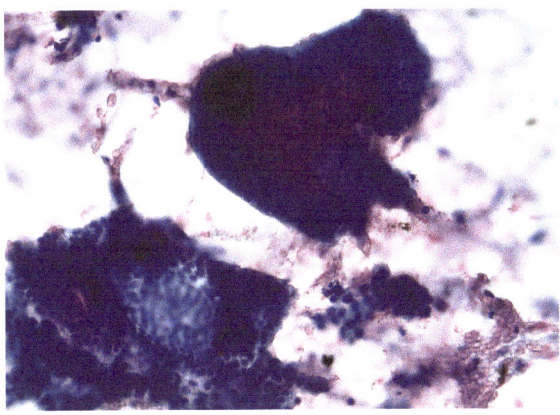

FIGURE 4.39. Adenoid cystic carcinoma. The aspirate harvested two large fragments of carcinoma consisting of tightly arranged uniform basaloid cells. A large refractile globule is evident in the fragment at 7 o'clock. (Smear, Papanicolaou.)

Pitfalls and Differential Diagnosis

- Sometimes difficult to distinguish from cribriform carcinoma of the breast
- Infiltrating lobular carcinoma
- Immunohistochemistry may be of some value in this distinction because cribriform breast carcinoma is usually estrogen and progesterone positive while adenoid cystic carcinoma is estrogen and progesterone negative
- Other mimics may be collagenous spherulosis and pleomorphic adenoma

## *Squamous Cell Carcinoma*

Clinical Features

- This entity should include only lesions that are predominantly squamous and not adenocarcinoma with squamous metaplasia.
- No specific clinical features of squamous cell carcinoma distinguish it from other subtypes.
- Squamous cell carcinoma may be a component of metaplastic carcinoma or may exist as a pure form.
- Approximately 10%–15% of pure squamous cell carcinomas have axillary node metastasis.

Cytomorphologic Characteristics (Figures 4.40 and 4.41)

- Cellular aspirate
- May be composed entirely of squamous cells, which are keratinizing, nonkeratinizing, or spindled
- Background keratinous debris and extensive necrosis
- Cystic degeneration and hemorrhage

Pitfalls and Differential Diagnosis

- Cytologic appearance of the aspirate may be identical in cases of primary breast squamous cell carcinoma versus metastatic squamous cell carcinoma. Clinical history plays a key role in the distinction of the former from the latter.

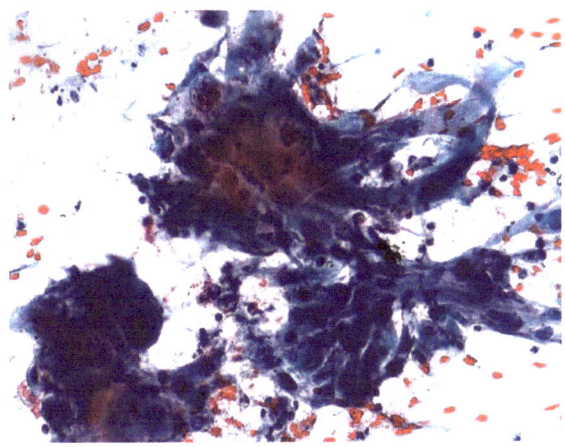

FIGURE 4.40. Squamous cell carcinoma. Poorly differentiated carcinoma with an irregular fragment of pleomorphic malignant cells with irregular, large, hyperchromatic nuclei. Squamous differentiation was more evident in other areas with keratinization. (Smear, Papanicolaou.)

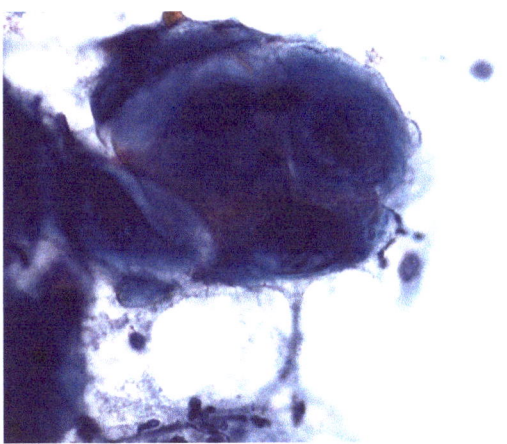

FIGURE 4.41. Squamous cell carcinoma. Higher magnification of a group of malignant cells with pleomorphic nuclei and macronucleoli. Note the well-defined cytoplasmic junctions, the only evidence of squamous differentiation in this case. (Smear, Papanicolaou.)

## *Inflammatory Carcinoma*

Clinical Features

- Inflammatory carcinoma refers to a particular form of breast carcinoma with an unusual presentation.
- Most cases have a prominent dermal lymphatic infiltration by tumor cells.
- The reported frequency of inflammatory carcinoma ranges from 1% to 10%.
- The age distribution is similar to that of ductal carcinoma NOS.
- Common clinical findings include diffuse erythema, induration, warmth, tenderness, edema, and, occasionally, a palpable mass.

Cytomorphologic Characteristics

- There is no significant inflammatory cell infiltrate.
- The inflammatory presentation is due to edema, which is the result of lymphatic obstruction by the tumor cells.
- The underlying infiltrating carcinoma has no specific features and is similar to poorly differentiated ductal carcinoma NOS
- There is usually low cellularity because of the edema. On-site evaluation is imperative to ensure an adequate sample for diagnosis.
- Cells occur singly or in loose clusters.
- There is fine cytoplasmic vacuolization.
- Pleomorphic nuclei with macronucleoli are present.
- Tumor diathesis occurs.

Pitfalls and Differential Diagnosis

- Acute mastitis/abscess
- Pregnancy/lactational changes

# Glycogen-Rich, Clear Cell Carcinoma

Clinical Features

- Glycogen-rich, clear cell carcinoma is a rare variant of invasive breast carcinomas, comprising 1%–3% of all breast carcinomas.
- The reported age ranges from 41 to 78 years, with a median age of 57 years.
- The clinical presentation is similar to ductal carcinomas NOS.
- This variant is considered to be more aggressive than the usual ductal carcinoma NOS, with an overall higher incidence of lymph node metastasis.

Cytomorphologic Characteristics

- The key histologic feature is the presence of neoplastic cells the majority of which have abundant clear cytoplasm containing glycogen.
- The neoplastic cells have sharp borders with clear or finely granular cytoplasm, which is periodic acid-Schiff positive and diastase labile.
- The nuclei are hyperchromatic, with prominent nucleoli.
- The hormone receptor status is similar to ductal carcinomas NOS.

Pitfalls and Differential Diagnosis

- Differential diagnosis of glycogen-rich, clear cell carcinomas includes other "clear cell tumors" such as lipid-rich carcinoma, clear cell hidradenoma, adenomyoepithelioma, and metastatic renal cell carcinomas.
- Ancillary studies including the use of immunohistochemistry are of immense value in avoiding diagnostic pitfalls.

# Apocrine Carcinoma

Clinical Features

- Pure apocrine carcinoma of the breast is rare, accounting for 0.3%–4% of all breast carcinomas.

- By World Health Organization definition, apocrine carcinoma should show cytologic and immunohistochemical characteristics of apocrine cells in greater than 90% of tumor cells.
- Apocrine carcinoma occurs in the older age group, more commonly in the sixth and seventh decades.
- The carcinoma probably arises from preexisting apocrine metaplasia rather than de novo.
- The prognostic significance of apocrine carcinoma is controversial. It is not any different from invasive mammary carcinomas NOS, although some reports suggest a somewhat better prognosis for this variant.
- Bilateral apocrine carcinomas are rare.

Cytomorphologic Characteristics (Figures 4.42 and 4.43)

- Hypercellularity is present.
- Sheets, cords and tubules, and single cells are loosely cohesive, often with prominent apocrine morphology.

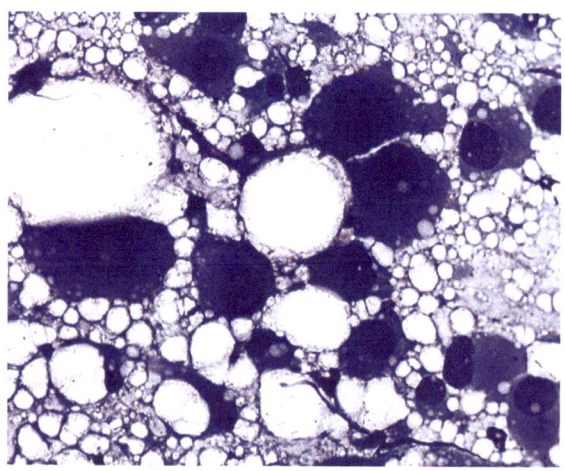

FIGURE 4.42. Apocrine carcinoma. A dispersed population of large, pleomorphic cells with polygonal shapes, large nuclei, and abundant granular cytoplasm. (Smear, Diff-Quik.)

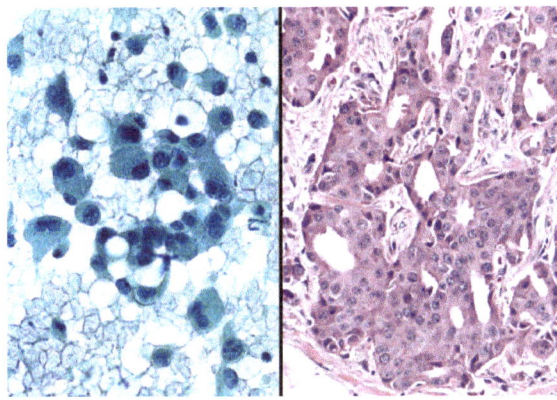

FIGURE 4.43. Apocrine carcinoma. A loosely cohesive cluster of large, pleomorphic malignant cells. Note the occasional binucleation and abundant granular cytoplasm in the tumor on the left. The corresponding histologic section is shown on the right. (Smear, Papanicolaou; histologic section, hematoxylin and eosin.)

- Cytologic evidence of malignancy is often easy to appreciate (nuclear overlap, pleomorphism, high nucleus to cytoplasm ratios, occasional mitoses).
- Pleomorphic large nuclei are often eccentrically located within the dense granular or clear eosinophilic cytoplasm. Cells are often binucleated with discrete and well-delineated cytoplasmic borders.
- The nucleoli are prominent, and multinucleation is common.
- Background consists of fragmented cytoplasm with naked malignant nuclei and granular debris.
- Eccentric nuclear placement gives the cells a "cometlike" morphology.
- Occasionally necrosis and/or histiocytes are seen.
- It represents one of the gray zone cytopathologic diagnoses on FNA.
- In difficult cases, immunostaining with Ki-67 (higher expression) and p53 can be helpful.

Pitfalls and Differential Diagnosis

- Atypical squamous metaplasia. This is an uncommon but a known cause of "atypical/suspicious" diagnosis on FNA. It shows moderate cellularity with syncytial sheets of atypical ductal cells with oval nuclei, coarse chromatin, angulated macronucleoli, and abundant amphophilic cytoplasm. There is often anisonucleosis and occasional bizarre cells with giant nucleoli. Apocrine differentiation is not readily apparent. Signet-ring forms have also been reported. Histologically, atypical squamous metaplasia is characterized by the replacement of ductal epithelium by a single layer of apocrine cells that display at least a threefold variation in nuclear size. "Atypical apocrine hyperplasia" is a similar lesion with hyperplastic features regarded by some as a form of atypical ductal hyperplasia. Additionally, atypical apocrine cells have also been reported on FNA in the setting of sclerosing adenosis (atypical apocrine adenosis). Although diagnostic confusion with ductal carcinoma NOS or apocrine carcinoma may arise on FNA, it is helpful to remember that, unlike carcinoma, in atypical squamous metaplasia the atypical nuclei are only focally present and are never a diffuse feature. Also many myoepithelial cells are present and no mitoses or karyorrhexis is noted. The true malignant potential of atypical squamous metaplasia is not known.
- Ductal carcinoma with neuroendocrine differentiation.
- Acinic cell carcinoma.
- Squamous cell carcinoma.
- Granular cell tumor.
- Metastatic tumors (malignant melanoma).
- Apocrine carcinoma arising in axillary apocrine glands should be distinguished from breast primaries.

## *Metaplastic Carcinoma*

Clinical Features

- Metaplastic carcinomas account for less than 1% of all invasive breast carcinomas.

- This extremely rare type of breast tumor includes various subtypes, that is, adenosquamous carcinoma, carcinosarcoma (homologous or heterologous), and spindle cell carcinomas.
- Tumors may be a monophasic (spindle cells only) or biphasic sarcomatoid type (carcinomatous and sarcomatous components).
- Clinical presentation is not different from the usual infiltrating breast carcinomas.
- These tumors may be cystic in nature.
- These tumors usually are very aggressive tumors with a poor prognosis.

Cytomorphologic Characteristics (Figures 4.44 to 4.46)

- Depends on the specific subtype
- May show an admixture of malignant glandular and squamous epithelium
- Spindle cells, with fusiform nuclei and delicate wispy cytoplasmic processes
- Occasional metachromatic stromal fragments
- Occasional multinucleated giant cells and malignant heterologous tumor elements
- Occasional necrotic and inflammatory debris in the smear background

Pitfalls and Differential Diagnosis

- Benign mixed tumor of the skin
- Sarcomas
- Squamous metaplasia in cystic lesions
- Metastatic cancers
- Phyllodes tumor
- Fibromatosis
- Nodular fasciitis

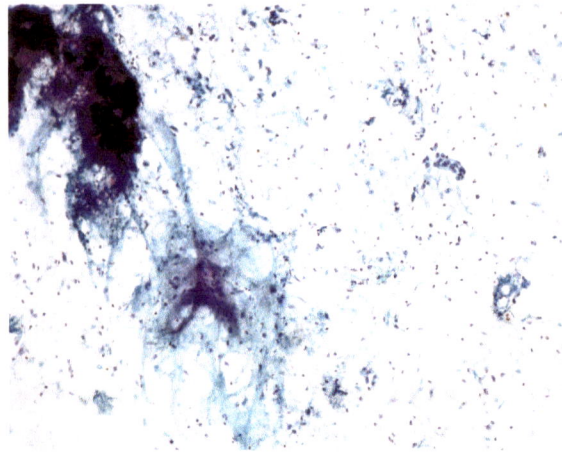

FIGURE 4.44. Metaplastic carcinoma. A hypercellular smear with numerous dissociated and spindled cells in a myxoid background. The cytopathologic appearance of this rare tumor can often be deceptively bland. (Smear, Papanicolaou.)

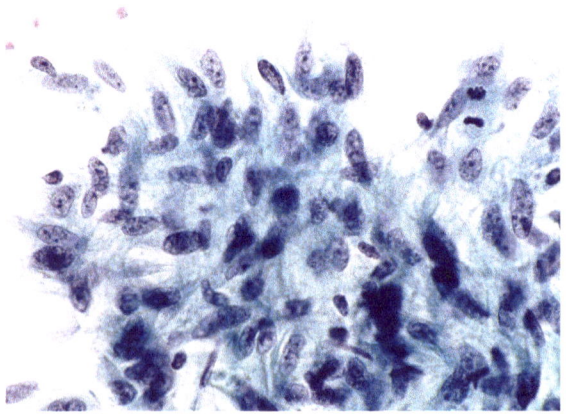

FIGURE 4.45. Metaplastic carcinoma. Higher magnification of the sarcomatoid variant displaying somewhat uniform mesenchymal-type cells with fusiform nuclei. Note the blunt nuclear edges and the mitotic figures. (Smear, Papanicolaou.)

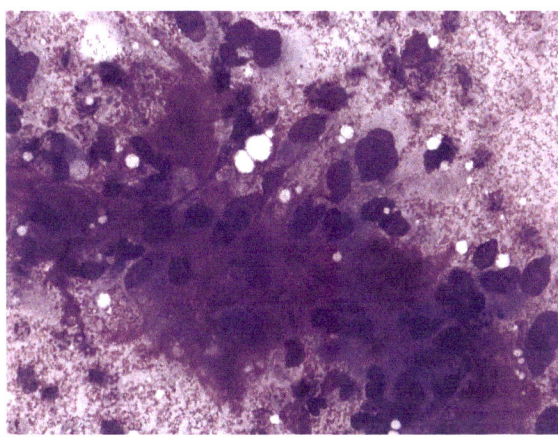

FIGURE 4.46. Metaplastic carcinoma. A dispersed population of pleomorphic malignant cells appearing as naked nuclei embedded within a granular, myxoid background. This myxoid stroma should not be confused with the biphasic appearance of a fibroadenoma. (Smear, Diff-Quik.)

## Carcinoma With Osteoclastic-Type Giant Cells

Clinical Features

- This is a rare variant of high-grade ductal carcinoma NOS and is characterized by the presence of osteoclastic giant cells in the stroma.
- A majority of the reported cases had lymph node metastasis, with a 5-year survival rate approaching 70%, similar to patients with ordinary infiltrating breast carcinomas.
- The giant cells are present in the stroma and are associated with an inflammatory, fibroblastic response with extravasated red blood cells, lymphocytes, and monocytes.
- The giant cells are histiocytic in origin as confirmed by positive staining for CD68 (KP-1) using immunohistochemistry. The histiocytic nature of these giant cells has also been confirmed by ultrastructural studies.

Cytomorphologic Characteristics (Figure 4.47)

- Hypercellular smears
- Osteoclastlike giant cells admixed with carcinoma cells

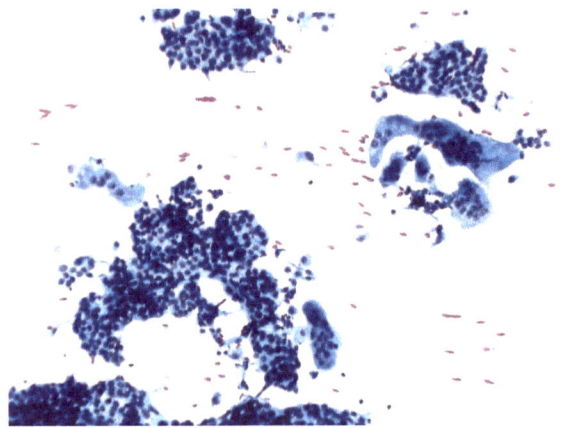

FIGURE 4.47. Carcinoma with osteoclastlike giant cells. Irregular fragments of pleomorphic carcinoma containing numerous multinucleated giant cells resembling osteoclasts. (Smear, Papanicolaou.)

Pitfalls and Differential Diagnosis

- Fibrocystic changes, papillomatosis

## Neuroendocrine Carcinoma

Clinical Features

- Primary neuroendocrine carcinomas of the breast are rare variants of infiltrating breast carcinoma.
- Neuroendocrine carcinoma represents 2%–5% of all invasive breast carcinomas.
- Most cases present in the sixth to seventh decade of life.
- Neuroendocrine tumors do not present any differently than other tumor types.
- Most patients present with a palpable mass.
- On mammography, the tumor nodule is well-circumscribed.
- In general, this type has a very poor prognosis.
- Neuroendocrine tumors include solid neuroendocrine carcinomas, small cell carcinomas, and large cell neuroendocrine carcinomas.

- This group of tumors is similar to neuroendocrine tumors of the lung and the gastrointestinal tract.
- Metastatic neuroendocrine carcinomas are more common than primary breast tumors of the same type, and lung is the most common source.
- Infiltrating breast carcinomas NOS may have focal endocrine differentiation and are not included in this group of primary neuroendocrine carcinomas.

Cytomorphologic Characteristics (Figure 4.48)

- Hypercellular
- Small round blue cells, uniformly lacking pleomorphism, arranged in a loosely cohesive fashion
- Nuclear molding, hyperchromasia, inconspicuous nucleoli, fine powdery chromatin, karyorrhexis, mitoses, and often nuclear crush artifact
- Cytopathologic distinction between primary and metastatic neuroendocrine carcinoma not possible on the aspirate

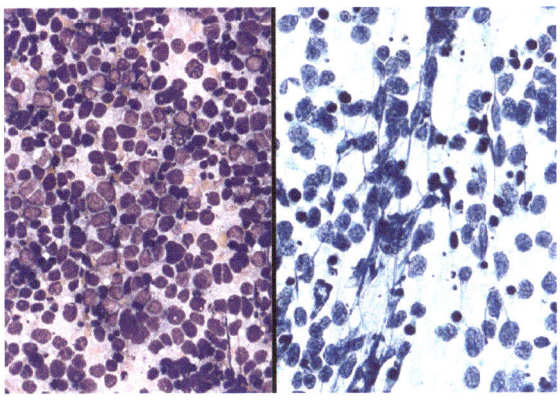

FIGURE 4.48. Neuroendocrine carcinoma. Hypercellular smear with singly dispersed carcinoma cells with high nucleus to cytoplasm ratios, nuclear hyperchromasia, and finely dispersed chromatin. Note the lymphocytelike morphology on Diff-Quik staining **(left)**. Also evident is nuclear crush artifact and numerous karyorrhectic nuclei **(right)**. (Smear, Diff-Quik and Papanicolaou, Diff-Quik.)

Pitfalls and Differential Diagnosis

- An important differential diagnosis to consider is a metastatic carcinoid or small cell carcinoma from another site.
- Immunohistochemical stains, other than neuroendocrine markers, may be utilized to distinguish between primary neuroendocrine carcinoma and small cell carcinoma from a metastatic tumor.
- In general, breast small cell carcinomas are CK-7 positive and CK-20 negative, whereas lung small cell carcinomas tend to be negative for CK7 and CK-20.
- In addition, estrogen and progesterone receptors and GCDFP-15 are positive in the primary breast carcinomas.
- To distinguish breast small cell carcinoma from infiltrating lobular carcinomas, E-cadherin may be of significant value.
- A majority of small cell carcinomas will be E-cadherin positive as compared with lobular carcinomas, which will all be negative.
- The neuroendocrine nature of these tumors can be confirmed by using neuroendocrine markers such as synaptophysin and chromogranin.

# Sweat Gland (or Salivary Gland-Type) Tumors

Clinical Features

- These are rare skin neoplasms (approximately 1 in every 20,000 skin malignancies).
- They rarely occur in the breast.
- Among the sweat gland carcinomas, those of eccrine origin are most common.
- Eccrine carcinomas may arise de novo from any portion of the normal eccrine apparatus or may result from the transformation of an existing benign eccrine tumor.
- Malignant hidradenoma is thought to originate from the distal eccrine excretory duct.

- They typically present as a solid or partially cystic nodule with a slight predilection for females of middle age.

Cytomorphologic Characteristics (Figures 4.49 and 4.50)

- Will depend on the type of sweat gland tumor. They may appear deceptively bland, basaloid, squamous, or mucinous. Accurate distinction from a primary ductal neoplasm could be extremely difficult on a limited FNA sample, particularly when a good clinical history and physical findings are not available at the time of FNA interpretation.

Pitfalls and Differential Diagnosis

- Primary breast carcinoma
- Metastatic carcinomas

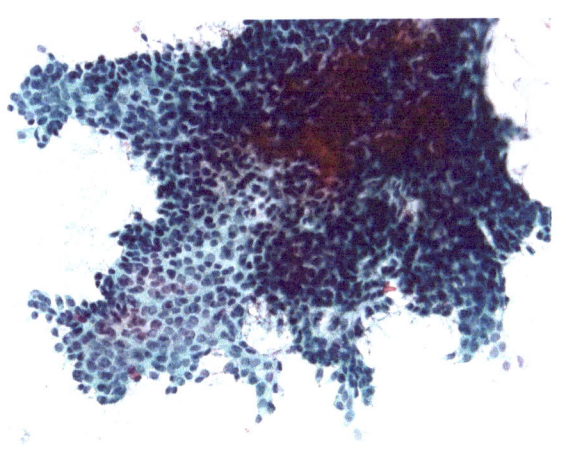

FIGURE 4.49. Sweat gland tumor (malignant nodular hidradenoma). A large epithelial fragment composed of round, uniform nuclei. A distinction from atypical ductal hyperplasia or well-differentiated ductal carcinoma can be difficult. However, note the absence of any single epithelial cells in the background. (Smear, Papanicolaou.)

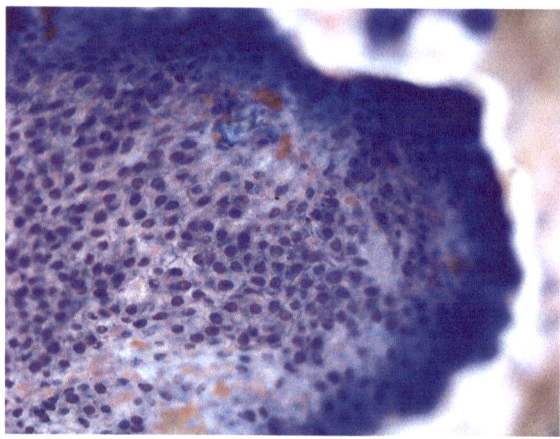

FIGURE 4.50. Sweat gland carcinoma (malignant nodular hidrade-noma). A higher magnification of cohesive epithelial fragments displays clear cytoplasm, uniform round nuclei, and well-defined polygonal cytoplasmic borders. These tumors have a low-grade morphology on fine-needle aspiration and can be quite challenging if adequate information of the physical findings is not available to the cytopathologist. (Smear, Diff-Quik.)

## Sarcomas of the Breast

Sarcomas of the breast comprise a variety of types and are rare, accounting for not more than 1% of all primary breast neoplasms. The sarcomas include angiosarcoma, leiomyosarcoma, stromal sarcoma, osteosarcoma, and liposarcoma. The clinical presentations of these entities are often variable. The following is a brief description of some of the more common primary sarcomas of the breast.

Angiosarcoma

*Clinical Features*

- Angiosarcomas of the breast are rare entities, comprising less than 0.05% of all primary malignancies of the breast.

- There are three forms of breast angiosarcomas: (1) primary angiosarcomas, (2) secondary angiosarcomas related to lymphedema due to mastectomy, and (3) secondary angiosarcomas related to radiation therapy following surgery.
- Angiosarcomas can be histologically graded into a three-tiered system: grade I (well-differentiated), grade II (intermediate differentiation), and grade III (poorly differentiated).
- Immunostains for factor VIII, CD34, and CD31 are helpful in characterizing the endothelial differentiation.

*Cytomorphologic Characteristics*

- Sparse cellularity, often blood-stained smears
- Single round to spindled hyperchromatic cells with prominent nucleoli
- Collagenized stroma
- Hemosiderin-laden macrophages, fibrin, necrosis
- May contain branching vessels in "tangles"

*Pitfalls and Differential Diagnosis*

- "False negativity" can be caused by scant cellularity and abundant blood.
- Atypical hemangioma of the breast may mimic an angiosarcoma.
- Radiotherapy-related changes may have overlapping cytologic features.
- Resolving hematoma/granulation tissue may also have similar cellular contents and may also be blood stained, mimicking the appearance of an angiosarcoma.

Malignant Phyllodes Tumor (Cystosarcoma Phyllodes)

Cystosarcoma phyllodes is an uncommon malignant tumor with heterogeneous morphology consisting of both epithelial and stromal elements. The cellularity and character of its stromal component is the most important feature distinguishing it from fibroadenoma. Only a small percentage (<10%) of phyllodes tumors are histologically overtly malignant.

*Clinical Features*

- Rare tumors, less than 1% of all breast tumors
- Initially present as discrete palpable masses that may show rapid enlargement

*Cytomorphologic Characteristics*

- Variable

*Pitfalls and Differential Diagnosis*

- Variable

Leiomyosarcoma

*Clinical Features*

- These primary smooth muscle tumors of the breast are rare, comprising less than 1% of all breast tumors.
- They arise most commonly from the smooth muscle of the nipple and areola.
- Leiomyosarcomas arise within the breast as well. Both present as slowly growing, palpable masses that may be painful.

*Cytomorphologic Characteristics*

- Variable cellularity
- Dissociated cells with sheets of spindle and round cells
- Increased mitotic activity, prominent nuclear atypia, and necrosis

*Pitfalls and Differential Diagnosis*

- Phyllodes tumor
- Metaplastic carcinoma
- Hemangiopericytoma
- Fibromatosis

# *Selected Reading*

Cai G, Simsir A, Cangiarella J: Invasive mammary carcinoma with osteoclast-like giant cells diagnosed by fine-needle aspiration biopsy: review of the cytologic literature and distinction from other mammary lesions containing giant cells. Diagn Cytopathol 2004, 30:396–400.

Cangiarella J, Waisman J, Shapiro RL, Simsir A: Cytologic features of tubular adenocarcinoma of the breast by aspiration biopsy. Diagn Cytopathol 2001, 25:311–315.

Dawson AE, Mulford DK: Fine needle aspiration of mucinous (colloid) breast carcinoma. Nuclear grading and mammographic and cytologic findings. Acta Cytol 1998, 42:668–672.

Gomez-Aracil V, Mayayo E, Azua J, Arraiza A: Papillary neoplasms of the breast: clues in fine needle aspiration cytology. Cytopathology 2002, 13:22–30.

Greeley CF, Frost AR: Cytologic features of ductal and lobular carcinoma in fine needle aspirates of the breast. Acta Cytol 1997, 41:333–340.

Gupta RK: Cytodiagnostic patterns of metaplastic breast carcinoma in aspiration samples: a study of 14 cases. Diagn Cytopathol 1999, 20:10–12.

Howell LP, Kline TS: Medullary carcinoma of the breast. An unusual cytologic finding in cyst fluid aspirates. Cancer 1990, 65:277–282.

Jain S, Gupta S, Kumar N, Sodhani P: Extracellular hyaline material in association with other cytologic features in aspirates from collagenous spherulosis and adenoid cystic carcinoma of the breast. Acta Cytol 2003, 47:381–386.

Jayaram G, Swain M, Chew MT, Yip CH: Cytologic appearances in invasive lobular carcinoma of the breast. A study of 21 cases. Acta Cytol 2000, 44:169–174.

Joshi A, Kumar N, Verma K: Diagnostic challenge of lobular carcinoma on aspiration cytology. Diagn Cytopathol 1998, 18: 179–183.

Kalogeraki A, Garbagnati F, Santinami M, Zoras O: E-cadherin expression on fine needle aspiration biopsies of breast invasive ductal carcinomas and its relationship to clinicopathologic factors. Acta Cytol 2003, 47:363–367.

Kumar PV, Talei AR, Malekhusseini SA, Monabati A, Vasei M: Papillary carcinoma of the breast. Cytologic study of nine cases. Acta Cytol 1999, 43:767–770.

Lamb J, McGoogan E: Fine needle aspiration cytology of breast in invasive carcinoma of tubular type and in radial scar/complex sclerosing lesions. Cytopathology 1994, 5:17–26.

Layfield LJ, Dodd LG: Cytologically low grade malignancies: an important interpretative pitfall responsible for false negative diagnoses in fine-needle aspiration of the breast. Diagn Cytopathol 1996, 15:250–259.

Levine PH, Waisman J, Yang GC: Aspiration cytology of cystic carcinoma of the breast. Diagn Cytopathol 2003, 28: 39–44.

McKee GT, Tambouret RH, Finkelstein D: Fine-needle aspiration cytology of the breast: Invasive vs. in situ carcinoma. Diagn Cytopathol 2001, 25:73–77.

Moroz K, Lipscomb J, Vial LJ, Jr., Dhurandhar N: Cytologic nuclear grade of malignant breast aspirates as a predictor of histologic grade. Light microscopy and image analysis characteristics. Acta Cytol 1997, 41:1107–1111.

Ng WK, Kong JH: Significance of squamous cells in fine needle aspiration cytology of the breast. A review of cases in a seven-year period. Acta Cytol 2003, 47:27–35.

Ng WK, Poon CS, Kong JH: Fine needle aspiration cytology of ductal breast carcinoma with neuroendocrine differentiation. Review of eight cases with histologic correlation. Acta Cytol 2002, 46:325–331.

Park IA, Ham EK: Fine needle aspiration cytology of palpable breast lesions. Histologic subtype in false negative cases. Acta Cytol 1997, 41:1131–1138.

Pettinato G, Pambuccian SE, Di Prisco B, Manivel JC: Fine needle aspiration cytology of invasive micropapillary (pseudopapillary) carcinoma of the breast. Report of 11 cases with clinicopathologic findings. Acta Cytol 2002, 46:1088–1094.

Rajesh L, Dey P, Joshi K: Fine needle aspiration cytology of lobular breast carcinoma. Comparison with other breast lesions. Acta Cytol 2003, 47:177–182.

Rogers LA, Lee KR: Breast carcinoma simulating fibroadenoma or fibrocystic change by fine-needle aspiration. A study of 16 cases. Am J Clin Pathol 1992, 98:155–160.

Saqi A, Mercado CL, Hamele-Bena D: Adenoid cystic carcinoma of the breast diagnosed by fine-needle aspiration. Diagn Cytopathol 2004, 30:271–274.

Sohn JH, Kim LS, Chae SW, Shin HS: Fine needle aspiration cytologic findings of breast mucinous neoplasms: differential diagnosis between mucocelelike tumor and mucinous carcinoma. Acta Cytol 2001, 45:723–729.

Stanley MW, Tani EM, Skoog L: Metaplastic carcinoma of the breast: fine-needle aspiration cytology of seven cases. Diagn Cytopathol 1989, 5:22–28.

Taniguchi E, Yang Q, Tang W, Nakamura Y, Shan L, Nakamura M, Sato M, Mori I, Sakurai T, Kakudo K: Cytologic grading of invasive breast carcinoma. Correlation with clinicopathologic variables and predictive value of nodal metastasis. Acta Cytol 2000, 44:587–591.

Tse GM, Ma TK: Fine-needle aspiration cytology of breast carcinoma with endocrine differentiation. Cancer 2000, 90:286–291.

Wong NL, Wan SK: Comparative cytology of mucocelelike lesion and mucinous carcinoma of the breast in fine needle aspiration. Acta Cytol 2000, 44:765–770.

Yu GH, Cajulis RS, De Frias DV: Tumor cell (dys)cohesion as a prognostic factor in aspirate smears of breast carcinoma. Am J Clin Pathol 1998, 109:315–319.

# 5
# Metastatic and Secondary Tumors

Metastatic and secondary tumors are uncommon in the breast (0.5%–2%) compared with primary neoplasms, but an accurate diagnosis on FNA is imperative for a definitive and rapid diagnosis, preceding the often nonsurgical treatment of these cases. The most common of these include malignant melanoma, non-Hodgkin lymphoma, and carcinomas of the lung, urogenital tract, and gynecologic tract. However, almost every known tumor has been seen metastatic to the breast and can create real diagnostic problems not only for the treating physicians and radiologists but also for pathologists when these lesions are aspirated. Radiologically (mammographically or on ultrasound), these lesions appear as single, round, discrete, and often large nodule or mass usually lacking the irregularities and microcalcifications of primary breast cancer.

It is therefore critical in view of a known history or in the face of an unusual cytomorphology during an on-site evaluation of a breast aspirate that additional material should be procured and triaged for the appropriate studies, including flow cytometry, immunoperoxidase studies, molecular genetics, and electron microscopy. If on-site evaluation is not possible, attempts should be made to obtain sufficient material to prepare a cell block and/or cytospin slides for ancillary studies.

# Hematologic Tumors: Malignant Lymphoma and Plasma Cell Tumors

## *Clinical Features*

- Malignant lymphomas of the breast, both primary and secondary, are extremely rare and may appear at any age.
- Patient may have multiple lesions, with up to 10% of patients presenting with bilateral disease.
- The clinical presentation may mimic primary breast carcinomas.
- Most often, primary and secondary lymphomas or plasma cell tumors may appear as well-circumscribed lesions of varying sizes.
- Lymphoma including Hodgkin lymphoma of the breast is commonly seen as a manifestation of a known generalized lymphoma and presents no difficulty in rendering a diagnosis.
- However, rarely they may occur as a primary breast cancer, with the majority of them being diffuse large B cell lymphomas.
- Immunophenotyping with immunocytochemistry or flow cytometry can establish the diagnosis.
- Axillary node involvement is seen in more than one third of the patients with lymphoma.
- Plasmacytomas of the breast are rare and generally present as circumscribed masses that appear solid by imaging.

## *Cytomorphologic Characteristics*
(Figures 5.1 to 5.5)

- Characteristics depend on the type of hematologic cancer; compare with a sample from a known primary.
- Reed-Sternberg cells are diagnostic of Hodgkin disease.

## *Pitfalls and Differential Diagnosis*

- Consider neuroendocrine carcinoma.
- Consider invasive lobular carcinoma.

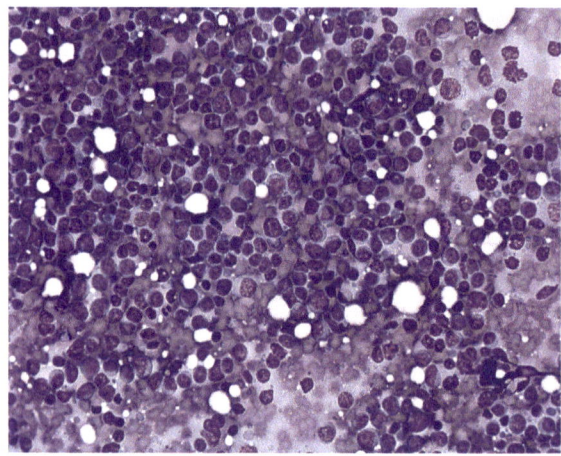

FIGURE 5.1. Non-Hodgkin lymphoma. Hypercellular smear with atypical monomorphic large lymphocytes. Few mitotic figures are also visible. Nuclei show prominent nucleoli, and a few mitotic figures are also noted. (Smear, Diff-Quik.)

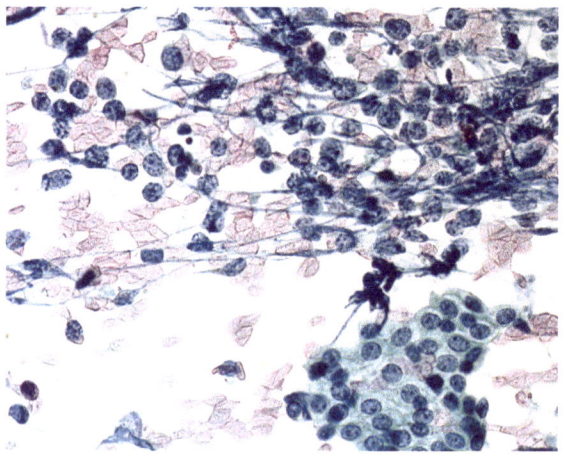

FIGURE 5.2. Non-Hodgkin lymphoma. Large malignant lymphocytes with prominent crush artifact and occasional mitotic figures. A partially intact fragment of benign ductal epithelium is noted in the lower right. (Smear, Papanicolaou.)

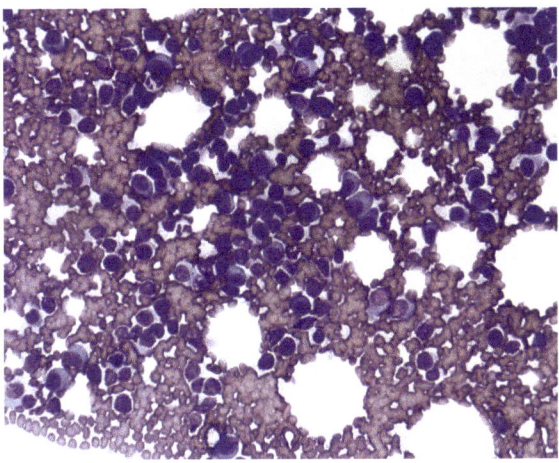

FIGURE 5.3. Plasmacytoma. A dissociated population of small round cells with predominance of mature-appearing plasma cells. Infiltrating ductal carcinoma composed of dispersed malignant cells may resemble a plasma cell neoplasm due to eccentric nuclear placement in the cells. (Smear, Diff-Quik.)

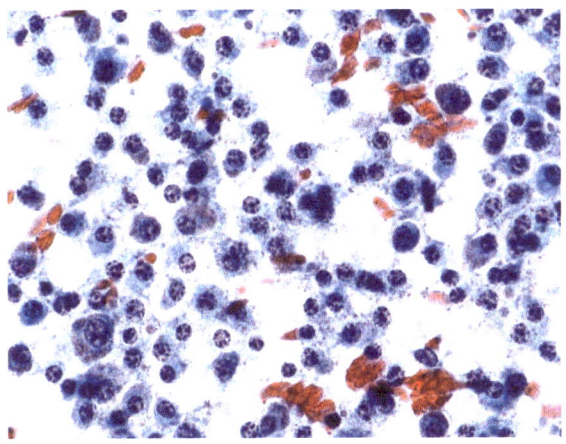

FIGURE 5.4. Plasmacytoma. This aspirate was obtained from the upper outer quadrant of the breast of a male patient with no prior history. The characteristic speckled "clock face" chromatin is obvious. (Smear, Papanicolaou.)

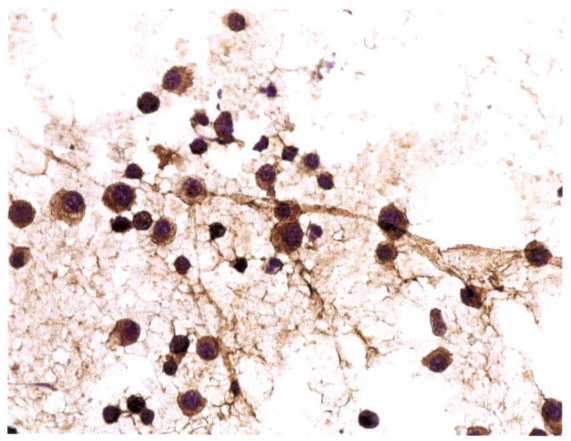

FIGURE 5.5. Plasmacytoma. Tumor cells show strong immunoreactivity with kappa light chain. (Smear.)

- Consider metastatic cancers.
- Plasmacytomas should be distinguished from plasma cell mastitis or amyloid tumors.
- Benign entities such as an intramammary lymph node with lymphoid hyperplasia may cause diagnostic difficulties.
- Immunohistochemistry and ancillary techniques such as flow cytometry are critical tools for arriving at a correct diagnosis.

# Metastatic Tumors

## *Clinical Features*

- Breast is an uncommon site for metastatic disease, and a history of another primary tumor is often not available (i.e., occult metastasis).
- Metastatic disease to the breast ranges from 0.5% to 6% of all breast malignancies, most commonly affecting women.

- The most common metastasis is from the contralateral breast.
- Virtually any malignancy may metastasize to the breast.
- The most common metastatic tumors of the breast are lung and malignant melanoma followed by ovary, kidney, thyroid, cervix, stomach, and prostate.
- In children and adolescents, rhabdomyosarcoma represents a common source of metastatic disease.
- Metastasis from other sites has also been reported.
- In men, prostate cancer is the most common form of metastatic tumor to the breast.
- Tumors are usually well circumscribed and freely mobile in the deep breast tissue.
- They are rarely predominantly cystic masses.
- Metastatic tumors may be multinodular and bilateral.
- Clinically, radiologically, and cytopathologically, metastatic tumors may mimic primary breast carcinomas.
- Sarcomas can also occur as a primary breast carcinoma or a metastasis from the other sites.
- Axillary lymph nodes are frequently involved.
- The most common locations for metastatic tumors are in the upper outer quadrant.
- Microcalcifications are extremely rare in metastatic breast carcinomas and have been described rarely in cases of metastatic carcinomas of ovarian origin produced by psammoma bodies.

## Cytomorphologic Characteristics
(Figures 5.6 to 5.15)

- Characteristics depend on the type of primary tumor.
- Usually the aspirates from metastatic tumors present with rich cellularity.
- If the cytomorphologic appearance is not that of a primary breast carcinoma, other diagnostic possibilities including metastatic disease must be entertained.

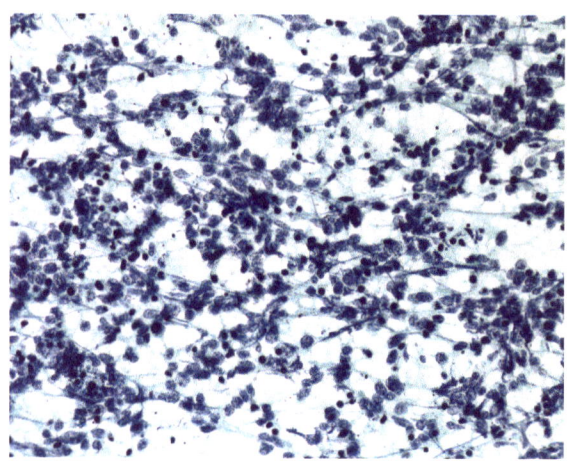

FIGURE 5.6. Metastatic small cell carcinoma of the lung. Hypercellular smear illustrating the characteristic neuroendocrine cytomorphology, that is, small round oval nuclei, fine dusty chromatin, nuclear molding, nuclear crush artifacts, and numerous karyorrhectic nuclei. Distinction from a primary neuroendocrine carcinoma of the breast is not possible on morphology alone. (Smear, Papanicolaou.)

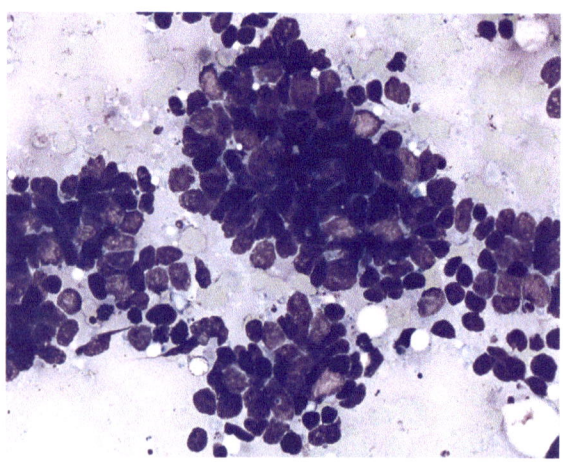

FIGURE 5.7. Metastatic small cell carcinoma of the uterine cervix. This patient in advanced clinical stage presented with a breast mass. Cytomorphology as seen here looks concordant with a primary cervical tumor. The smear is hypercellular with large nests of neuroendocrine cells, depicting high-grade morphology. Note prominent nuclear molding, lack of cytoplasm, and abundant karyorrhexis. (Smear, Diff-Quik.)

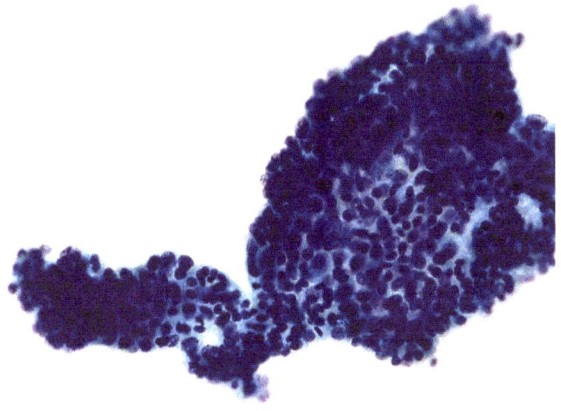

FIGURE 5.8. Metastatic papillary serous carcinoma of the ovary. This patient had a known ovarian primary at the time of aspiration. Note the papillary arrangement of this large tissue fragment. Cytomorphologic distinction from primary breast papillary carcinoma is not possible on morphology. (Smear, Papanicolaou.)

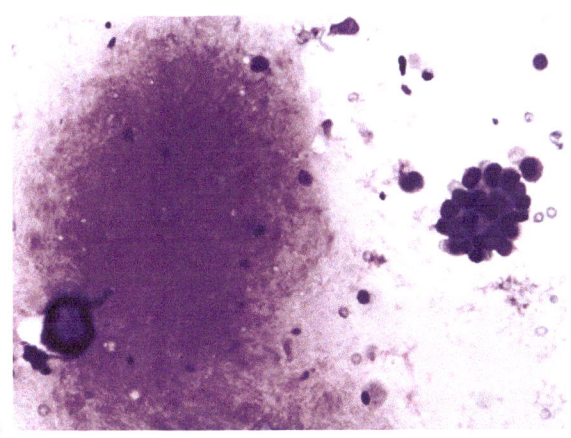

A

FIGURE 5.9. **(A)** Metastatic papillary serous carcinoma of the ovary. A single psammoma body is evident at 8 o'clock, along with a three-dimensional tissue fragment and abundant cystic debris. (Smear, Diff-Quik.)

(Continued)

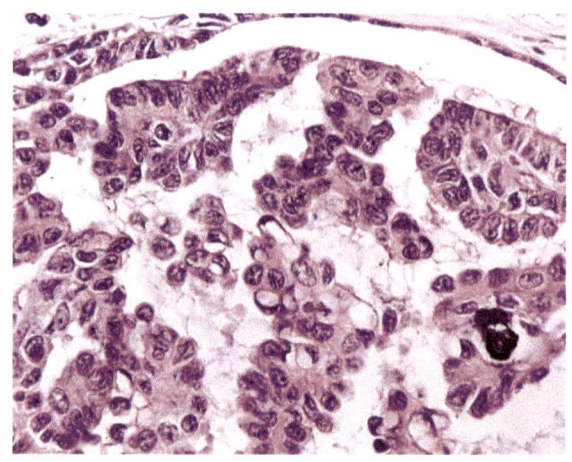

B

FIGURE 5.9. **(B)** Metastatic papillary serous carcinoma of the ovary. Histologic section of the corresponding tumor shows a well-developed papillary architecture with associated psammoma bodies. (Hematoxylin and eosin.)

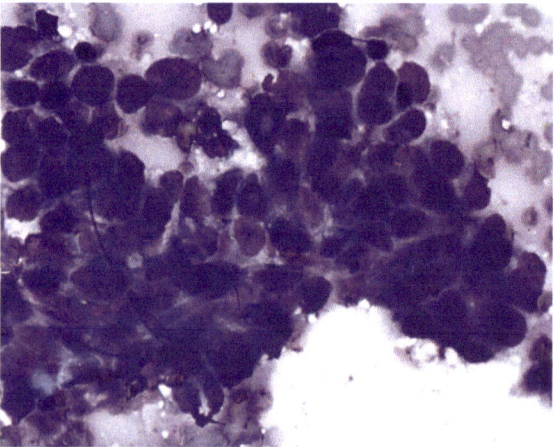

FIGURE 5.10. Metastatic medullary thyroid carcinoma. An irregular fragment of pleomorphic malignant cells with high nucleus to cytoplasm ratios and prominent pleomorphism and anisonucleosis. A rare intranuclear inclusion is seen toward the center. There is nothing in this smear to suggest a medullary carcinoma diagnosis. Clinical history and immunoperoxidase staining are crucial when dealing with metastasis in the breast. (Smear, Diff-Quik.)

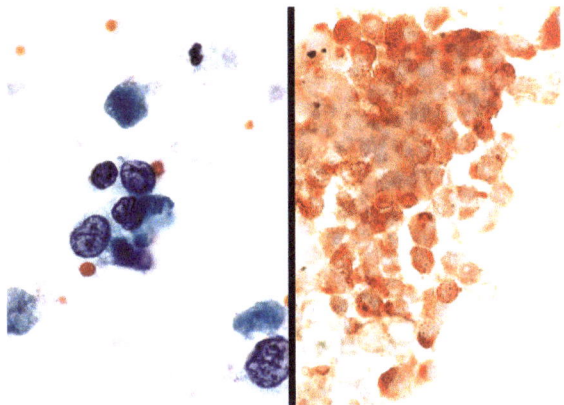

FIGURE 5.11. Metastatic medullary thyroid carcinoma. Note the isolated tumor cells with naked nuclei associated with fragments of amorphous material consistent with amyloid **(left)**. An immunostain for calcitonin is strongly positive **(right)**. (Smear, Papanicolaou.)

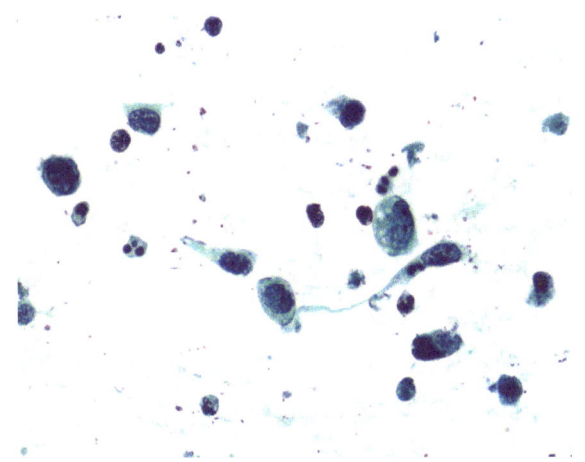

FIGURE 5.12. Metastatic malignant melanoma. Isolated, singly placed pleomorphic malignant cells. Note prominent anisonucleosis and long tapering cytoplasmic tails. Metastatic melanoma can closely mimic primary breast carcinoma and is not an uncommon metastasis to the breast. (Smear, Papanicolaou.)

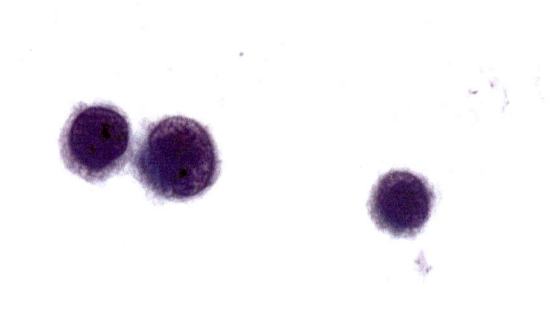

FIGURE 5.13. Metastatic malignant melanoma. This case presented as a cystic breast mass and on aspiration revealed rare single malignant cells resembling histiocytes and inflammatory cells. (Smear, Papanicolaou.)

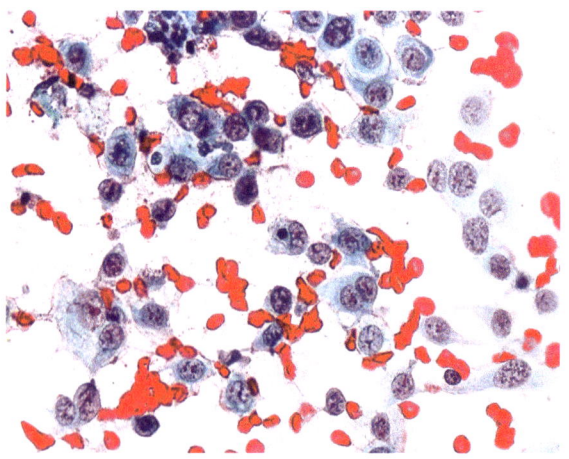

FIGURE 5.14. Metastatic malignant melanoma. Note the prominent epithelioid morphology of the malignant cells with round to oval nuclei and macronucleoli. Cells also show frequent binucleation. (Smear, Papanicolaou.)

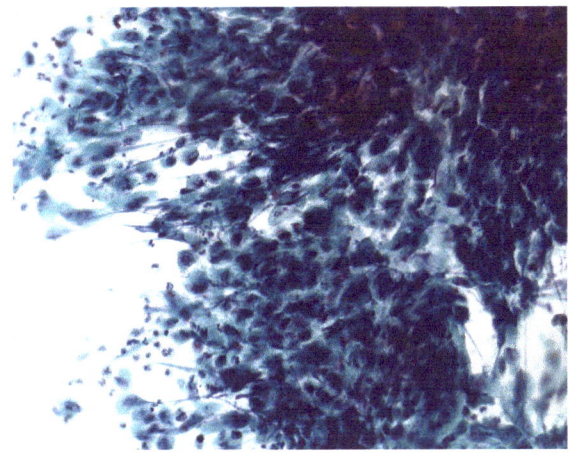

FIGURE 5.15 Metastatic squamous cell carcinoma of the lung. The carcinoma is poorly differentiated and shows large syncytial tissue fragments. No keratinization is evident. (Smear, Papanicolaou.)

- Based on the site of the origin of the tumor, the aspirates may present with various cell types, including pleomorphic and spindle shapes, with varying sizes and cellular arrangements.
- Some of the metastatic tumors may resemble primary breast tumors such as squamous, clear cell, or mucinous carcinomas.
- Malignant melanoma (see Figures 5.12 to 5.14), squamous cell carcinoma (see Figure 5.15), various adenocarcinomas, and pleomorphic sarcomas exhibit a pleomorphic population of large cells.
- Melanoma, lymphoma, leukemia, and poorly differentiated carcinomas present with a dispersed cell pattern.
- Malignant melanoma cells may contain pigment and/or intranuclear inclusions and they can be bi- or multinucleated (see Figures 5.12 to 5.14).
- Neuroendocrine tumors and small cell carcinoma of the lung present with small-sized tumor cells (see Figure 5.6 and 5.7).

- Spindle cell tumors often represent various types of sarcomas.
- The aspirates of sarcomas are cellular usually with a spindle cell pattern.
- Electron microscopy and immunostaining for mesenchymal markers are helpful to establish the diagnosis of a sarcomatous lesion.

## Pitfalls and Differential Diagnosis

- It is critical to distinguish between a primary breast carcinoma versus metastatic disease because of the varied differences in therapeutic approaches and the differences in the patients' outcome.
- Even though the clinical presentation of the two may be very similar, in general, nipple discharge and retraction are not usually seen in metastatic tumors.
- Metastatic tumors have variable mammographic features ranging from features similar to peripheral breast disease, cyst or fibroadenoma to those of a malignant lesion such as medullary carcinoma.
- Microcalcifications are not frequent except in rare cases of psammoma bodies in metastatic tumors of ovary or thyroid.
- Usually the patients with metastatic breast lesions experience a poor outcome, and about 80% of them die within 1 year.
- It is important to appreciate that the distinction between a primary breast tumor versus a metastasis may not always be possible on the basis of a fine-needle aspirate or even a core biopsy specimen.
- The initial and a very crucial step in diagnosis of a metastatic breast lesion is the recognition of a cytologic pattern that is not the usual presentation of a primary breast carcinoma.
- This should alert the cytopathologist to explore the possibility of a metastasis.

- Once again, a careful review of clinical history and the pathology slides of the original primary tumor may help elucidate this process.
- The judicial use of a panel of immunohistochemistry stains and ancillary studies such as electron microscopy and flow cytometry may also be helpful.
- Useful immunostains include hormonal receptors such as estrogen and progesterone and GCFDP-15; positive results from such stains generally are helpful to classify the lesion as a primary breast tumor.
- An immunochemical panel that repeats the one performed on the primary tumor can also identify a metastatic lesion if the panel results are comparable.

## Selected Reading

Akcay MN: Metastatic disease in the breast. Breast 2002, 11:526–528.

Cangiarella J, Symmans WF, Cohen JM, Goldenberg A, Shapiro RL, Waisman J: Malignant melanoma metastatic to the breast: a report of seven cases diagnosed by fine-needle aspiration cytology. Cancer 1998, 84:160–162.

Cangiarella J, Waisman J, Cohen JM, Chhieng D, Symmans WF, Goldenberg A: Plasmacytoma of the breast. A report of two cases diagnosed by aspiration biopsy. Acta Cytol 2000, 44:91–94.

David O, Gattuso P, Razan W, Moroz K, Dhurandhar N: Unusual cases of metastases to the breast. A report of 17 cases diagnosed by fine needle aspiration. Acta Cytol 2002, 46:377–385.

Domanski HA: Metastases to the breast from extramammary neoplasms. A report of six cases with diagnosis by fine needle aspiration cytology. Acta Cytol 1996, 40:1293–1300.

Ewing CA, Miller MJ, Chhieng D, Lin O: Nonepithelial malignancies mimicking primary carcinoma of the breast. Diagn Cytopathol 2004, 31:352–357.

Filie AC, Simsir A, Fetsch P, Abati A: Melanoma metastatic to the breast: utility of fine needle aspiration and immunohistochemistry. Acta Cytol 2002, 46:13–18.

Levine PH, Zamuco R, Yee HT: Role of fine-needle aspiration cytology in breast lymphoma. Diagn Cytopathol 2004, 30:332–340.

Singh NG, Kapila K, Dawar R, Verma K: Fine needle aspiration cytology diagnosis of lymphoproliferative disease of the breast. Acta Cytol 2003, 47:739–743.

Sneige N, Zachariah S, Fanning TV, Dekmezian RH, Ordonez NG: Fine-needle aspiration cytology of metastatic neoplasms in the breast. Am J Clin Pathol 1989, 92:27–35.

# 6
# Breast Ductal Lavage

To obtain *nipple aspiration fluid* (NAF), a pump and/or a syringe connected to a suction cup is applied to the nipple and the aspirated fluid is collected using a capillary tube. This procedure yields NAF in 59%–99% of women. A volume of 20–30 µl of fluid can be obtained (range 1–200). About 77% of the cells of NAF are foam cells of macrophage derivation, and only 13% are ductal epithelial cells (median 120 cells/duct). Criteria for evaluation of NAF were developed in the mid-1970s and are similar to the criteria used for evaluation of breast FNA material. The cytologic findings in NAF from 2,701 volunteer women with no family history of breast cancer and no breast carcinoma at the time of enrollment were analyzed prospectively. The overall incidence of breast cancer in this cohort was 4.4% after median follow-up of 12.7 years. In this study, both incidence and relative risk of breast cancer increased with increasing severity of cytologic diagnosis of the NAF (Table 6.1). Although the relative risk of breast cancer associated with abnormal NAF was reduced in an updated analysis of the data, these results have generated much interest in the use of mammary cytology for the evaluation of breast cancer risk.

Some investigators have detected in NAF factors associated with mammary neoplasia; others have performed proteomic analysis and molecular evaluation of NAF, but there is no clinical application for these findings at present.

TABLE 6.1. Nipple aspiration fluid cytology and breast cancer: prospective evaluation of nipple aspiration fluid in 2,343 women, with average follow-up of 12.7 years.

| Cytologic diagnosis | Women with breast cancer/women with same diagnosis | Percent with breast cancer | Adjusted relative risk |
|---|---|---|---|
| No breast fluid | 9/352 | 2.6 | 1.0 |
| Unsatisfactory | 15/315 | 4.8 | 1.4 |
| Normal | 56/1,291 | 4.3 | 1.8 |
| Hyperplasia | 18/327 | 5.5 | 2.5 |
| Atypical hyperplasia | 6/58 | 10.3 | 4.9 |
| Total | 104/2,343 | 4.4 | |

Low volume, paucity of epithelial cells, and abundance of degenerative changes constitute limitations to the use of NAF. Ductal lavage has been developed to obviate these problems.

*Ductal lavage* (DL) is a minimally invasive procedure that allows in vivo sampling of the ductal epithelium. A microcatheter is inserted in a fluid-yielding nipple duct, followed by lavage with 10–20 mL of saline solution in 2- to 4-mL increments; the lavage fluid is then collected, and the cytology of the epithelial cells is examined. In a study comparing NAF and DL samples obtained from a cohort of 507 women at high risk of breast cancer, DL yielded samples with greater number of ductal cells than NAF (Table 6.2). In the same study, both NAF and DL identified two patients with

TABLE 6.2. Characteristics of samples obtained by nipple fluid aspiration and ductal lavage.

| | Nipple aspiration fluid (417 women) | Ductal lavage (383 women) |
|---|---|---|
| Epithelial cells/duct | 120 (Range 10–74,300) | 13,500 (Range 43–492,000) |
| Satisfactory samples | 27% | 78% |
| Mild atypia | 27 (6%) | 66 (17%) |
| Marked atypia | 12 (3%) | 24 (6%) |
| Malignant | 2 (<1%) | 2 (<1%) |

undiagnosed carcinoma, but the number of DL cases with abnormal cytology (mild and marked atypia) was more than fourfold higher than for NAF (see Table 6.2). Some investigators have proposed the use of DL for breast cancer risk assessment, but no data are available at present to guide the clinical application of this novel technique.

For historical reasons, micropore filter preparations of DL (and NAF) samples were obtained in the feasibility study, but liquid-based preparations and cytospin slides can also be used. In the feasibility study, only 10 epithelial cells per duct were required for a satisfactory DL specimen, to allow correlation with prior results. Because DL yields at least 10-fold more epithelial cells than NAF, a higher number of cells should be required for a satisfactory DL sample. Nonetheless, even the presence of abundant epithelium does not guarantee that a DL sample will be representative of the alterations in the duct.

The criteria used for evaluation of DL cytology are similar to those used for breast FNA. Direct comparison of DL and FNA samples obtained from the same cases of carcinoma underscores the morphologic similarities between the two types of sample. Cell arrangement, cell size, nuclear size and size variation, nuclear membrane irregularity, chromatin granularity, and presence of large nucleoli are the cytologic features most helpful in the identification of abnormal epithelial cells in DL samples.

*Benign ductal cells* (Figures 6.1 to 6.3) are usually present in flat sheets and clusters of less than three cell layers. They are small and uniform in size, with rare and small nucleoli. Myoepithelium is present admixed with the benign ductal cells.

In a*typical ductal cells* (Figures 6.4 to 6.10), *mild atypia* is defined by the presence of ductal cells with slight nuclear enlargement. The epithelium is organized in monolayers, small clusters, and single cells. The nuclear membrane is smooth, the nuclear chromatin is finely granular, and small nucleoli are present.

Ductal cells with *marked atypia* can be present singly, in monolayers, or in small clusters; large clusters of more than

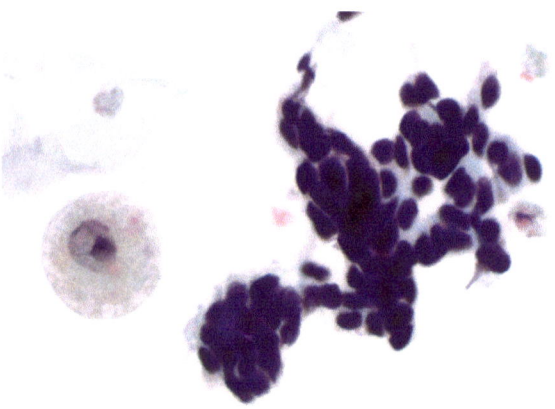

FIGURE 6.1. Benign ductal cells, uniform in size, with indistinct cell borders, can be arranged in clusters of fewer than three cell layers. Note the small size of nuclei in relation to that of a macrophage. (Thin Prep®, Papanicolaou.)

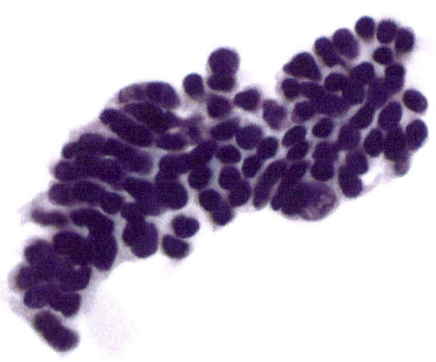

FIGURE 6.2. A cohesive cluster of benign ductal cell with honeycomb arrangement. (Thin Prep®, Papanicolaou.)

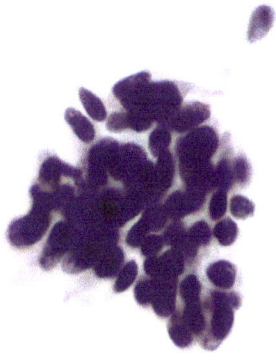

FIGURE 6.3. Benign ductal cells in a pseudopapillary tridimensional group (less than three cell layers). Nuclei are slightly enlarged, but regularly spaced and uniform. Rare and inconspicuous nucleoli may be seen. (Thin Prep®, Papanicolaou.)

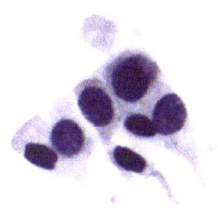

FIGURE 6.4. A flat but dyshesive cluster of atypical ductal cells, with enlarged nuclei and evident nucleoli. (Thin Prep®, Papanicolaou.)

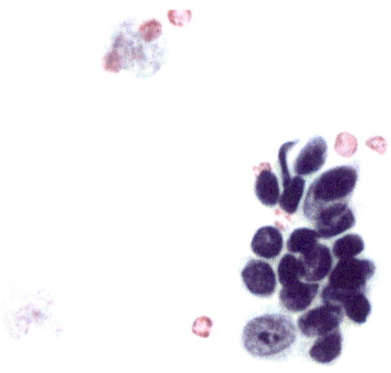

FIGURE 6.5. A dyshesive tridimensional cluster of atypical ductal cells, with enlarged nuclei and evident nucleoli. (Thin Prep®, Papanicolaou.)

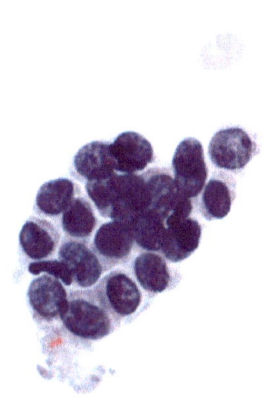

FIGURE 6.6. A dyshesive tridimensional cluster of atypical ductal cells, with admixed myoepithelium. This "ball-like" configuration correlated with lobular carcinoma in situ in the surgical tissue specimen. (Thin Prep®, Papanicolaou.)

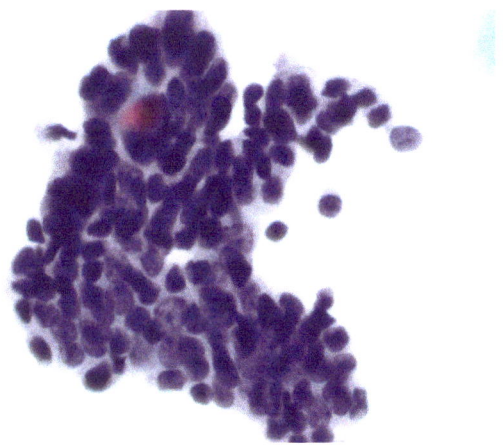

FIGURE 6.7. A cohesive cluster of atypical ductal cells, showing crowded and irregular honeycomb arrangement, enlarged nuclei, and noticeable nucleoli. (Thin Prep®, Papanicolaou.)

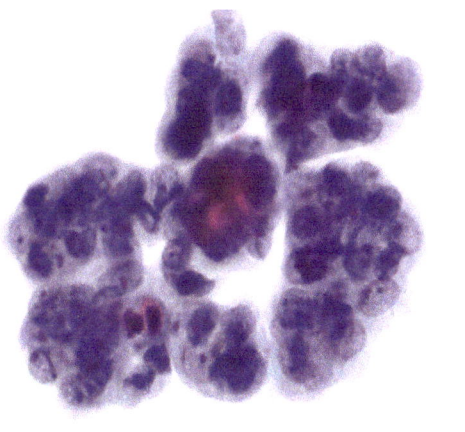

FIGURE 6.8. Papillary clusters of markedly atypical ductal cells, with nuclear enlargement, hyperchromasia, and prominent nucleoli. (Thin Prep®, Papanicolaou.)

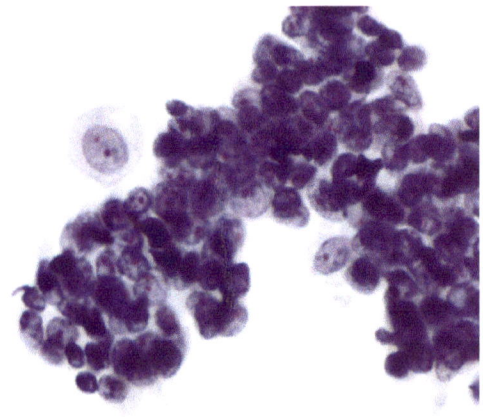

FIGURE 6.9. A cluster of markedly atypical ductal cells, with more than three cell layers, crowded and enlarged nuclei, nuclear hyperchromasia, and nucleoli. (Thin Prep®, Papanicolaou.)

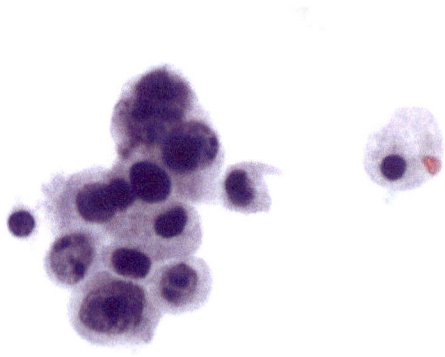

FIGURE 6.10. A dyshesive cluster of markedly atypical ductal cells with apocrine morphology. Anisonucleosis, nuclear hyperchromasia, and irregular nuclei are noted. (Thin Prep®, Papanicolaou.)

two cell layers are found in half of the cases. These cells show disorderly arrangement, moderate to marked nuclear enlargement, with high nuclear to cytoplasm ratio, nuclear overlap and anisonucleosis, irregular nuclear membrane, and coarse chromatin. Multinucleated cells and mitoses can also be present. Calcifications occur in about half of cases with marked atypia, but necrotic debris is rare.

*Neoplastic cells* in DL specimens show the characteristic features of malignancy. In our experience, the number of malignant cells is also a determinant in rendering a definitive diagnosis of malignancy.

Ljung and collaborators speculate that the diagnostic category of "mild atypia" encompasses the spectrum of changes of usual ductal hyperplasia and atypical ductal hyperplasia, whereas "marked atypia" corresponds to a spectrum of changes from atypical ductal hyperplasia to ductal carcinoma in situ. However, information from clinical follow-up studies is required and not yet available to support (or disprove) this statement.

Reproducibility in diagnosis of DL samples in time and among different observers is a requisite for clinical application of the technique. High agreement (kappa >0.70) among two reviewers from the same laboratory was reported for characteristics of nuclear size, anisonucleosis, nucleoli, mitoses, and necrosis. In another study, interobserver agreement among three reviewers from different laboratories was fair to good (kappas 0.6, 0.5, and 0.48), and mild atypia was the least reproducible diagnosis. Johnson-Maddux and colleagues have reported low reproducibility in the diagnosis of mild atypia in DL samples obtained from the same patient after a 6-month interval and have hypothesized that mild atypia might not be a correlate of epithelial dysplasia, but rather of hormonal status.

The findings in DL samples obtained from women undergoing mastectomy for carcinoma have been correlated with the histologic findings in the paired mastectomy specimen. In one study, dye injection through the microcatheter was used to identify the duct sampled by DL. Ducts involved by carcinoma in situ (ductal or lobular type) were identified in six cases, and ducts or lobules in tissue sections also containing carcinoma in situ were found in seven. These findings demonstrate that DL had sampled a duct involved by carcinoma in situ or an area of the breast spatially close to carcinoma in about 80% of cases. Nonetheless, DL has low sensitivity for the detection of carcinoma, and a benign sample cannot exclude malignancy. Khan et al. have obtained similar results and noted that the location of carcinoma in situ in relation to the nipple may affect the ability to detect atypical cells in the DL fluid. In both studies, the results of DL in the cancer-affected breast may have been limited due to possible distortion of the ducts caused by invasive carcinoma in some cases.

Lobular carcinoma in situ, an alteration of the mammary epithelium associated with high risk of breast carcinoma, was the only morphologic alteration in three mastectomy specimens in one correlative study. Two of the corresponding DL samples showed mild atypia with morphologic features compatible with lobular carcinoma in situ. Injected blue dye identified a duct and a few lobules involved by lobular carcinoma in situ in one case. This is, to date, the only documented example of DL sampling lobular carcinoma in situ.

Because of some limitations in the cytologic interpretation of DL samples, future evaluation of this type of sample may combine cytology with other techniques, such as methylation-specific polymerase chain reaction, analysis of loss of heterozygosity, chromosome copy number determination, and/or proteomic analysis.

Studies are in progress to investigate the clinical significance of the new methodologies summarized in this chapter. "Intraductal" investigation of mammary carcinoma and its precursor lesions can provide insight into the biology of this disease and its clinical management. Cytology has had a determinant role in the development of this novel approach and will most certainly continue to play a critical role in their future development and application.

# Selected Reading

Brogi E, Miller MJ, Casadio C, Ljung B-M, Montgomery L: Paired ductal lavage and fine needle aspiration specimens from patients with breast carcinoma. Diagn Cytopathol 2005, 33: 370–375.

Brogi E, Robson M, Panageas KS, Casadio C, Ljung BM, Montgomery L: Ductal lavage in patients undergoing mastectomy for mammary carcinoma: a correlative study. Cancer 2003, 98: 2170–2176.

Dooley WC, Ljung BM, Veronesi U, Cazzaniga M, Elledge RM, O'Shaughnessy JA, Kuerer HM, Hung DT, Khan SA, Phillips RF, Ganz PA, Euhus DM, Esserman LJ, Haffty BG, King BL, Kelley MC, Anderson MM, Schmit PJ, Clark RR, Kass FC, Anderson BO, Troyan SL, Arias RD, Quiring JN, Love SM, Page DL, King EB: Ductal lavage for detection of cellular atypia in women at high risk for breast cancer. J Natl Cancer Inst 2001, 93:1624–1632.

Johnson-Maddux A, Ashfaq R, Cler L, Naftalis E, Leitch AM, Hoover S, Euhus DM: Reproducibility of cytologic atypia in repeat nipple duct lavage. Cancer 2005, 103:1129–1136.

Khan SA, Wiley EL, Rodriguez N, Baird C, Ramakrishnan R, Nayar R, Bryk M, Bethke KB, Staradub VL, Wolfman J, Rademaker A, Ljung BM, Morrow M: Ductal lavage findings in women with known breast cancer undergoing mastectomy. J Natl Cancer Inst 2004, 96:1510–1517.

King EB, Barrett D, King MC, Petrakis NL: Cellular composition of the nipple aspirate specimen of breast fluid. I. The benign cells. Am J Clin Pathol 1975, 64:728–738.

King EB, Barrett D, Petrakis NL: Cellular composition of the nipple aspirate specimen of breast fluid. II. Abnormal findings. Am J Clin Pathol 1975, 64:739–748.

King EB, Chew KL, Petrakis NL, Ernster VL: Nipple aspirate cytology for the study of breast cancer precursors. J Natl Cancer Inst 1983, 71:1115–1121.

King BL, Crisi GM, Tsai SC, Haffty BG, Phillips RF, Rimm DL: Immunocytochemical analysis of breast cells obtained by ductal lavage. Cancer 2002, 96:244–249.

Krassenstein R, Sauter E, Dulaimi E, Battagli C, Ehya H, Klein-Szanto A, Cairns P: Detection of breast cancer in nipple aspirate fluid by CpG island hypermethylation. Clin Cancer Res 2004, 10:28–32.

Krishnamurthy S, Sneige N, Ordonez NG, Hunt KK, Kuerer HM: Characterization of foam cells in nipple aspirate fluid. Diagn Cytopathol 2002, 27:261–265.

Ljung BM, Chew KL, Moore DH, 2nd, King EB: Cytology of ductal lavage fluid of the breast. Diagn Cytopathol 2004, 30:143–150.

National Cancer Institute: The uniform approach to breast fine-needle aspiration biopsy. National Cancer Institute Fine-Needle Aspiration of Breast Workshop Subcommittees. Diagn Cytopathol 1997, 16:295–311.

Sartorius OW, Smith HS, Morris P, Benedict D, Friesen L: Cytologic evaluation of breast fluid in the detection of breast disease. J Natl Cancer Inst 1977, 59:1073–1080.

Sauter ER, Ehya H, Schlatter L, MacGibbon B: Ductoscopic cytology to detect breast cancer. Cancer J 2004, 10:33–41; discussion 15–36.

Sauter ER, Ross E, Daly M, Klein-Szanto A, Engstrom PF, Sorling A, Malick J, Ehya H: Nipple aspirate fluid: a promising non-invasive method to identify cellular markers of breast cancer risk. Br J Cancer 1997, 76:494–501.

Wrensch MR, Petrakis NL, King EB, Miike R, Mason L, Chew KL, Lee MM, Ernster VL, Hilton JF, Schweitzer R, et al.: Breast cancer incidence in women with abnormal cytology in nipple aspirates of breast fluid. Am J Epidemiol 1992, 135:130–141.

Zhu W, Qin W, Ehya H, Lininger J, Sauter E: Microsatellite changes in nipple aspirate fluid and breast tissue from women with breast carcinoma or its precursors. Clin Cancer Res 2003, 9:3029–3033.

# Index

If you have any concerns about our products,
you can contact us on
**ProductSafety@springernature.com**

In case Publisher is established outside the EU,
the EU authorized representative is:
**Springer Nature Customer Service Center GmbH**
**Europaplatz 3, 69115 Heidelberg, Germany**

Printed by Libri Plureos GmbH
in Hamburg, Germany